THE REFERENCE SHELF     VOLUME 39   NUMBER 2

# NEW TRENDS IN THE SCHOOLS

### EDITED BY

## WILLIAM P. LINEBERRY

*Managing Editor, Foreign Policy Association*

THE H. W. WILSON COMPANY

NEW YORK        1967

# THE REFERENCE SHELF

The books in this series contain reprints of articles, excerpts from books, and addresses on current issues and social trends in the United States and other countries. There are six separately bound numbers in each volume, all of which are generally published in the same calendar year. One number is a collection of recent speeches; each of the others is devoted to a single subject and gives background information and discussion from various points of view, concluding with a comprehensive bibliography.

Subscribers to the current volume receive the books as issued. The subscription rate is $12 ($15 foreign) for a volume of six numbers. Single numbers are $3 each.

PRINTED IN THE UNITED STATES OF AMERICA

# PREFACE

American education has entered a period of great ferment. Innovations long in the talking stage are finally—and rapidly—moving into effect. An aura of excitement pervades the entire field, as the willingness and the wherewithal to experiment coupled with increasingly effective means for measuring results are stimulating a wide range of reforms. Today, a decade after Sputnik I first shattered our complacency, America's schools are alive with a welter of new ideas and programs so extensive in character that a compilation such as this can only scratch the surface and point to emerging trends.

An unprecedented influx of wealth and talent is largely responsible for this burgeoning activity. The seed-work of major institutions such as the Ford, Rockefeller, and Carnegie foundations has grown increasingly important. The reformist zeal of dedicated men like James Bryant Conant, whose critical study *The American High School Today* appeared just eight years ago and whose "second report," entitled *The Comprehensive High School,* has just been published, also has had a wide-ranging impact. And with the passage of the Elementary and Secondary Education Act of 1965, the awesome resources of the Federal Government have additionally been thrown into the fray. In fact, through civil rights enforcement and antipoverty funds alone, the Federal Government has become far and away the greatest catalyst for change in the history of our schools. Education, as President Lyndon B. Johnson has repeatedly emphasized, holds the key to the Great Society; and Americans at every level, from impoverished Negroes in our urban ghettoes to business and labor leaders active in the war on poverty, are emphatically making it clear that they agree.

The new trends being generated by these forces for change are as diverse as they are promising. No pat, all-encompassing educational philosophy stands behind the current ferment. Rather, the atmosphere is one of carefully researched and fi-

3

nanced experiment in a number of directions. New emphasis on individualized instruction goes forward at the same time that some cities erect huge, one-campus schools covering all grades from first through high school. Projects like the federally supported Head Start are designed to help culturally deprived children enter first grade with an opportunity for learning equal to that of their culturally advantaged classmates, while other programs are searching out brainpower and encouraging exceptional children to advance as fast as their capacities will allow.

Across the broad spectrum of education, new approaches and new techniques are coming into their own. The "new math" is already a fixture in many of the nation's school districts. The "new English" and the "new social studies" are clamoring for similar acceptance. And, as the last article in this compilation points out, technology—including those mind-stretching computers and their potential for programed instruction—is already knocking at the schoolhouse door.

This compilation is designed to acquaint the general reader with some of the salient new trends now under way in the schools. Not all of these trends have been enthusiastically welcomed in all quarters, nor have all of them necessarily lived up to expectations. For this reason, various critical articles are included where appropriate.

In the first section—a broad overview of the current educational scene—the backdrop against which reforms and innovations are taking place is reviewed. The reader may be interested to know how his state or region measures up to others in the task of educating its youth. The second section throws the spotlight on some of the forces working for reform—the need for fully developing our gifted children in our increasingly complex and demanding society, for example, and the need to shatter the dropout-delinquency syndrome. A major force for change—the Federal Government and its growing involvement in education—is given separate treatment in Section III.

Sections IV and V focus on the new trends themselves. Some recent innovations in vocational education, in gradeless schools, in huge, one-campus complexes, and in summer school are detailed in the former, while the latter concentrates on the revolution in methods that is sweeping so many of our school systems, with an extended look at the promise of the new technology.

The compiler wishes to thank the authors and publishers who have courteously granted permission for the reprinting of their materials in this book.

WILLIAM P. LINEBERRY

April 1967

## A NOTE TO THE READER

The reader's attention is directed to three recent Reference Shelf numbers also dealing with problems in American education: *America's Educational Needs* (Volume 30, Number 5), edited by Grant S. McClellan; *Federal Aid to Education* (Volume 33, Number 4), edited by Ronald Steel; and *Colleges at the Crossroads* (Volume 37, Number 6), edited by this compiler. Each of these compilations provides background for any reader interested in further pursuit of the subject.

# CONTENTS

PREFACE .............................................. 3

I. BACKGROUND TO A CHANGING ORDER

Editor's Introduction .................................... 9
Richard de Neufville and Caryl Conner. How Good Are Our
    Schools? ........................ American Education 10
The Widening Gap in Quality ......... Carnegie Quarterly 22
Harold Howe II. What's Wrong and Right—An Overview
    ............................... American Education 26
John Cogley. Catholic Schools and Their Problems ........
    .................................... Saturday Review 30

II. THE FORCES OF REFORM

Editor's Introduction .................................... 41
George C. Keller. The Search for "Brainpower" ...........
    ..................................... Public Interest 42
Edward T. Chase. The Waste of Manpower ...........
    .................................. Harper's Magazine 52
James S. Coleman. The Imbalance in Educational Opportunity
    ....................................... Public Interest 62
Schools as Social Instruments: A Critique ...............
    ......................... U.S. News & World Report 69

III. IMPACT OF THE FEDERAL GOVERNMENT

Editor's Introduction .................................... 77
Christopher Jencks. Washington Sponsors a Revolution ....
    ..................................... New Republic 78
The Elementary and Secondary Education Act of 1965: An
    Analysis ........................ American Education 87

Myron Lieberman. Civil Rights Enforcement ............
.................................. Phi Delta Kappan 100
Federal Pressures on the North .... U.S. News & World Report 110


IV. SOME RECENT INNOVATIONS

Editor's Introduction ................................... 115
James Nathan Miller. Vocational Education: A New Approach
...................................... PTA Magazine 116
Arthur D. Morse. Schools Without Grades ................. 122
Charles S. Carleton. Project Head Start: An Assessment ....
............................... American Education 132
One Campus for All Schools .... U.S. News & World Report 138
Benjamin H. Pearse. Making Summer School Count .......
............................... American Education 142


V. THE REVOLUTION IN METHODS

Editor's Introduction ................................... 150
Andrew Schiller. The Coming Revolution in Teaching English
................................. Harper's Magazine 151
Kenneth E. Brown and others. The New Math: A Progress
Report ......................... American Education 166
Charles E. Silberman. Applying the New Technology .....
.......................................... Fortune 176


BIBLIOGRAPHY .......................................... 198

# I. BACKGROUND TO A CHANGING ORDER

## EDITOR'S INTRODUCTION

How good are our schools? How do they measure up to the demands of our industrialized and specialized society, and what are their major defects? These are the questions that professional educators ask themselves year in and year out. They are the questions out of which reforms emerge.

The logical starting place for an examination of new trends in American education is a survey of the current school scene, with special attention to its outstanding problems. In many ways America's schools today must be judged inadequate to the times in which we live. Imbalance is a major problem. A vicious circle of poverty, poor teaching and poor facilities, and continued poverty entraps large segments of our population, particularly minority groups. Despite Federal efforts at equalization, money flows haphazardly to where, in socioeconomic terms, it is needed least and least to where it is needed most. At the same time, existing facilities are both overtaxed and underutilized. For selected hours of the day they are crammed with frantic activity, but for whole months of the year they stand virtually useless and empty. As the United States Commissioner of Education, Harold Howe II, points out: "The only buildings that are used less than the schools are the churches."

In other ways, too, our educational systems are beset by problems. The first article in this section points up some of these in a survey, state by state and region by region, of the scholastic performance of a broad selection of young men entering the armed forces. The failure rate of draftees helps to pinpoint both geographically and sociologically some failures in our schools. The second article details the plight, financial and otherwise, of our central city school districts, which face more problems, perhaps, than any others in the nation.

Next the United States Commissioner of Education draws a broad picture of our nationwide educational establishment in terms of both its failures and its achievements. Finally, John Cogley, former religious news editor of the New York *Times,* surveys the nation's Catholic schools and their problems. With one out of every seven children in the country now obtaining a parochial education, the special problems of these schools must inevitably demand attention in any survey of the current scene.

## HOW GOOD ARE OUR SCHOOLS? [1]

How good are our schools? How much do they teach our youngsters? Are schools in Maine as good as schools in California? Better? How do we tell?

Questions like these have become a pastime that threatens to supplant baseball as a national sport, says Helen Rowan, editor of *The Carnegie Quarterly.* The name of the game: How Good Are Our Schools? (Some players, notes Miss Rowan, prefer to call it How Bad Are Our Schools?) The rules are few: each player propounds his favorite opinion on education. He may say, "Kids learned to read better fifty years ago than they do today," or, "Northern schools are good and southern schools are lousy."

The beauty of it, continues Miss Rowan, is that anybody can win, since there is no way of proving or disproving the above or any similar assertion.

Miss Rowan's fancy is unfortunately close to truth. In the absence of meaningful information, public opinion about schools has rested largely on subjective judgment and popular impression.

While citizens debate, however, a number of Government agencies have been quietly stockpiling data that may bring the new game down for the count and leave baseball once again unchallenged.

By far the largest stockpiler of information is the Army's Office of the Surgeon General, which can tell us the following about some hypothetical young men:

[1] From article by Richard de Neufville, assistant professor of engineering, Massachusetts Institute of Technology, and Caryl Conner, managing editor of *American Education. American Education.* 2:1-7. O. '66. *American Education* is a publication of the United States Office of Education.

Joe Dangerfield and John Dangerfield are among approximately two million young men taking the Armed Forces Qualification Test (AFQT) and related examinations this year.

Both are eighteen and white. Yet, statistically Joe is eight times as likely to fail the tests as John. Why? John went to school in Washington. Joe went to school in Tennessee.

David Coldstream and Dick Coldstream are taking the same tests. Both are eighteen and Negro. David is three times as likely to fail the tests as Dick. David went to school in South Carolina; Dick in Rhode Island.

Bill Hardwood and Bob Hardwood will take the same tests. Both are eighteen. Bill is white and Bob is Negro. Both went to school in Florida. Bob is four times as likely to fail this test as Bill.

### Measuring Strengths and Weaknesses

What are the Armed Forces mental tests, and what do they have to do with schools?

The basic test in the Armed Forces is the AFQT. All draftees and enlistees are required to take it before entering any branch of the military services. It is a standard examination administered on a uniform basis throughout the country.

In the last ten years, over ten million young men aged eighteen to twenty-six have taken the AFQT. This is the largest group of standardized test scores that has ever been available for state and regional comparison.

For these reasons, these mental test results are the closest thing there is to a national index of educational strengths and weaknesses. Though the narrowness of range and the imprecision of scoring limit the test's usefulness for educators (it doesn't, for example, break down categories of information; it doesn't say that 40 per cent of failing eighteen-year-olds from Ohio were strong in math but weak in vocabulary), for the general public the AFQT and the related tests are the best available indicator of state-by-state school performance.

The absence of basic educational information is one of the odd phenomena of contemporary America. As a nation, we have developed highly sophisticated techniques to measure such disparate things as the purity of our water, the health of our economy, and the popularity of our public figures, but there has never been a measure of the basic academic skills of our children. We know the gross national product; we do not know the gross educational product.

When the Office of Education was established a century ago, Congress directed it to collect "such statistics and facts as shall show the condition and progress" of American education. Today the Office can accurately report the number of classrooms, teachers, pupils, books, globes, and language laboratories per pupil in every school in this country. But it doesn't know what students learn in these schools, or whether they learn it better or worse than students of fifty years ago. We know infinitely more about steel production in Pittsburgh, garment prices in Dallas, and the status of beef raising in Iowa than we do about the level of English or math proficiency anywhere in the Union. . . .

Whatever their value, tests have become an integral part of our statistic-happy American way of life. Colleges use them to determine admissions; industry uses them to make personnel decisions; TV programs use them to build ratings; party givers use them to entertain guests. The Armed Forces use the AFQT in connection with personnel assignment as well as in acceptance of draftees and enlistees.

Seymour L. Wolfbein, the former director of the Office of Manpower, Automation, and Training in the Department of Labor, called the AFQT "an excellent device for identifying persons with special educational and training problems." A report by the President's Task Force on Manpower Conservation called the AFQT "a uniform national test" which "has the potential for providing the communities of the nation with an important comparison and indicator . . . which would be difficult indeed to create if it did not already exist." Stafford L. Warren, former special assistant to the President for mental retardation, agreed on the great value of the AFQT as a means of identifying persons in need of special training.

## Value of the AFQT

The Army has used the experiences of half a century of testing in developing the AFQT, which, by law, is used to screen American youth for all branches of the Armed Forces. It follows a long line of other tests. In World War I, the Army Alpha (verbal) and Beta (nonverbal) tests were used. During World War II the Army used the AGCT (Army General Classification Test). The AFQT, designed and first used in 1950, has undergone frequent revision. The current versions cover, as have their predecessors since 1953, four subject areas: vocabulary, arithmetic, spatial relationships, and mechanical ability. There are twenty-five questions in each category. Questions are arranged in cycles of increasing difficulty in each of the four test areas. Fifty minutes are allowed. It is a "spiral omnibus" test emphasizing power rather than speed. The Army says it is not an intelligence test nor does it measure educational attainment as such, "although both education and intelligence affect the ability to score well on the test."

In general [says a report from the Surgeon General of the Army], there is a positive correlation between AFQT scores and education. The youth's score on the AFQT depends on several factors: on the level of his educational attainment, on the quality of his education (quality of his school facilities), and on the knowledge he gained from his educational training otherwise, in and outside of school. These are interrelated factors, which vary with the youth's socioeconomic and cultural environment, in addition to his innate ability to learn.

## Scoring

Raw scores on the AFQT are computed by subtracting one third of an examinee's mistakes from his total correct answers—a procedure adopted to compensate for lucky guesses. To supply meaning to the scoring and to simplify comparisons, the raw score is converted into a percentile score that theoretically establishes the examinee's relative standing in the whole draft-age population. (These relative standings are based on norms established a generation ago, during World War II. They have never been updated.) On the basis of this percentile score, men are classified into one of five mental groups:

| Mental group | Percentile score |
|:---:|:---:|
| I | 93-100 |
| II | 65- 92 |
| III | 31- 64 |
| IV | 10- 30 |
| V | 0- 9 |

Groups I, II, and III automatically meet mental standards for military service. (Some of these men are disqualified for medical reasons. Data in this article relate only to acceptance or rejection on the basis of mental tests scores. Total rejection rates are higher than those that appear here.)

Under the Universal Military Training and Service Act, men in mental Group V are considered unfit for military service unless their educational or occupational background seems to indicate that they should not have failed the test. In such cases there is a "terminal screening" and if its findings are at variance with the test score, the examinee is declared "administratively acceptable" and classified 1-A. (Last year [1965] about three thousand young men entered the Army this way.)

Procedures for Group IV vary according to the Army's manpower needs. Currently, all Group IV's who score above the sixteenth percentile *and have completed high school* are accepted for military service. All other men in Group IV take additional aptitude tests called the Army Qualification Battery (AQB). Failing scores on the AQB result in a "trainability limited" classification.

These men would qualify for military service only in time of war or national emergency.

(A new program just announced by Secretary of Defense Robert McNamara will take an additional group of men in mental Group IV [40,000 this year, 100,000 annually in subsequent years] and provide them with basic literacy training to enable them to qualify for military service. Precedent is the successful literacy training program conducted under Army auspices during World War II.). . .

## How the States Ranked

By now the Surgeon General's Office has accumulated enough data to provide a detailed state-by-state outline of successes and failures that reveals sharply uneven performance both by state and by race. The study of eighteen-year-olds, for example, shows that:

Failure rates on the AFQT and related tests ranged from a low of 6 per cent in the state of Washington to a high of 55 per cent in the District of Columbia. (The national average was 25 per cent.)

These rejection rates based on the mental tests are lowest in the midwestern and western states, highest in the South.

An unpublished supplement to the study, showing detail by race, reveals that:

Southern whites are behind whites in all other regions of the country; southern Negroes are behind Negroes in all other regions of the country.

In every state, test performance is significantly higher for whites than for Negroes. Nationally, only 19 per cent of the whites fail the mental tests, compared to a failure rate of 68 per cent for Negroes.

In addition, a special Department of Labor study of the academic background of 2,500 rejectees shows that:

Negroes who fail the AFQT average one more year of school than whites; characteristically they have had some high school experience while most white failures have not.

An examination of accumulated data on rejectees in the period from 1958 through 1965 supports findings from the study of eighteen-year-olds. Men from the western and midwestern states consistently performed best on the mental tests; men from the South consistently scored lowest. Throughout the eight-year period, moreover, the rank order of the states changed only slightly and the spread of percentage points between the states with the lowest failure rate averages (Washington, Iowa, Montana, Utah, Minnesota, Oregon) and those with the highest averages (Mississippi,

South Carolina, Louisiana, North Carolina, Alabama, Georgia) has remained about the same. . . .

The eight-year cumulative results for draftees differ only in minor detail from the results of the study of eighteen-year-olds. . . .

Over a long period of time, the draftee rejection rates more accurately reflect regional differences in performance by young men. But, by excluding enlistees, these figures exaggerate the inadequacy of national performance on the AFQT. Enlistees, prescreened by local recruiters before taking the test, seldom fail the AFQT. Since a majority of all men who enter the Armed Forces enter as enlistees, the over-all rejection rate (enlistees plus draftees) is substantially less than for draftees alone.

*Draftee Failure Rate (by per cent)*
*Fiscal Year 1966*

| *Army area* | *All* | *White* | *Negro* |
|---|---|---|---|
| III (South) | | | |
| Ala., Fla., Ga., Miss., N.C., S.C., Tenn. | 31 | 18 | 68 |
| IV (South Central) | | | |
| Ark., La., N.M., Okla., Tex. | 20 | 12 | 57 |
| I, II (Northeast) | | | |
| Conn., Maine, Mass., N.H., N.J., N.Y., R.I., Vt., Del., D.C., Ky., Md., Ohio, Pa., Va., W. Va. | 15 | 12 | 45 |
| V, VI (Midwest and West) | | | |
| Colo., Ill., Ind., Iowa, Kan., Mich., Minn., Neb., N.D., S.D., Wis., Wyo., Ariz., Calif., Idaho, Mont., Nev., Ore., Utah, Wash. | 10 | 8 | 37 |

(Source: Results of Preinduction Examination Summary. Office of the Surgeon General, Department of the Army.)

Failure rates clearly and consistently relate to geographical areas. Year after year, men from the West and the Midwest perform better than those from other parts of the country. In the special study of eighteen-year-olds, their failure rate was only half the national average, while men from the South were failing at twice the national rate.

The same regional differences appear in a study of draftee failures by race [indicated in the preceding table].

Throughout the United States the failure rate of whites on these examinations averages one fourth that of Negroes. The exception is West Virginia where whites and Negroes fail in equal—and substantial—numbers. In every other state the Negro failure rate is at least twice that of the white failure rate.

Among successful examinees—men who pass the tests—whites also do much better than Negroes. Fewer than one twentieth as many Negroes score in mental Group I as would be expected on the basis of the theoretical norms for the standard population. More than two thirds of the Negroes examined for military service in 1966 fell in Group IV or below. By theoretical distribution, 69 per cent would fall in Groups I, II, and III; less than 22 per cent of the Negroes did so. Specifically:

*Estimated Percentage Distribution of Draftees by Mental Group, by Race: Fiscal Year 1966*

| Mental group | White | Negro | Total |
|---|---|---|---|
| I | 7.6 | 0.3 | 6.7 |
| II | 32.1 | 3.3 | 28.8 |
| III | 34.6 | 18.2 | 32.8 |
| IV | 16.0* | 38.2* | 18.5* |
| V | 9.1 | 37.1 | 12.3 |
| Administratively acceptable | 0.6 | 2.9 | 0.9 |

* Mental group IV consists of (a) white—9.4% passed AQB, 6.6% failed AQB (trainability limited); (b) Negro—17.5% passed AQB, 20.7% failed AQB (trainability limited); (c) total —10.3% passed AQB, 8.2% failed AQB (trainability limited).

## *Impact of Poverty*

These test results mirror America's erratic progress toward its elusive goal of educational equality. They also reflect the host of disturbing social and economic problems that face the nation: For example, the 1963 Department of Labor study reported that the majority of young men failing the AFQT, white and Negro alike, were the products of poverty. Forty per cent of them had never gone beyond grammar school, four out of five didn't finish high school, almost one third came from broken homes, and one fifth came from families that have needed public assistance. The unemployment rate for rejectees was substantially higher than for other young men in the same age group, and most of those who were employed held unskilled jobs and had by far the lowest earnings in their age group.

Clearly this suggests a relationship between failing scores on the mental tests and the environment of poverty, just as the regional extremes point to a serious inequality of educational opportunity.

The most relevant index for appraising the quality of education in a community is the degree to which it provides the basic knowledge and skills that are required in our contemporary world. AFQT results tell a great deal more than the number of men who are not qualified intellectually to enter the Armed Forces. These same young men are equally unqualified to become contributing members of our work force. They have not been educated to provide for themselves and their families.

Today's military rejects include tomorrow's hard-core unemployed [said President John F. Kennedy]. The young man who does not have what it takes to perform military service is not likely to have what it takes to make a living.

The rejection rate on the AFQT is not an infallible guide, but it is impressive evidence of failure by many schools. The grown man who cannot pass the AFQT is in serious trouble. This test does not measure innate intelligence or scholastic aptitude—it measures precisely those skills that are most important in terms of jobs and income.

With rare exceptions, those who fail have had all the formal schooling they are going to get. Only 4 per cent of the rejectees the

Department of Labor studied in 1963 had taken business or commercial courses and only 17 per cent had taken vocational or technical courses. The substantial majority of rejectees had been in academic courses—but their most common deficiency on the AFQT was apparently that they could not read or do simple arithmetic.

The extreme variations in regional performance clearly suggest that schools have not erased inequality based on accidents of geography; the extreme racial variations make it clear that the schools have yet to overcome the environmental handicaps of the nation's Negro students. It is unlikely that the talent pool in any one state is substantially different than the talent pool in any other state. It is a demonstrable fact that the talent pool in any one ethnic group is substantially the same as that in any other ethnic group.

### The Failure of Our Schools

"There is absolutely no question of any genetic differential," says a special Department of Labor report on the Negro family. "Intelligence potential is distributed among Negro infants in the same proportion and pattern as among Icelanders or Chinese or any other group."

In every generation talent appears at every social stratum in every geographic area. "In every race, nation, class, and community, better and worse endowed individuals can be found," wrote anthropologist Juan Comas. "This is a biological fact to which there are no exceptions."

Thus the AFQT results seem to point up failure in the schools. Whatever the combination of nonschool factors—poverty, unstable families, community attitudes, low educational level of parents, etc. —which put minority group students at a disadvantage in verbal and nonverbal skills when they enter first grade, it is clear that the schools do not overcome them, notes a just-completed report by the United States Office of Education.

The OE report is based on a study of educational opportunity that included achievement testing of as many as 135,000 students at one of five way-points in their educational career—first, third, sixth, ninth, and twelfth grades. At each grade level the Negro pupils scored distinctly lower than did white students but most important to note is that by the twelfth grade the difference had *increased*.

For example, Negroes were 10.7 points below whites in non-verbal scores in the first grade. By twelfth grade this gap had grown to 11.1 points. In verbal scores, the gap widened from 7.2 points in first grade to 11.2 points by twelfth grade.

Thus, whatever the degree of inequality when the youngster enters the school system, it is greater when he leaves. The schools not only fail to close the gap, they don't even enable Negro students to hold their own.

The over-all differences mentioned should not obscure the fact that many Negro children outperform white children. Additionally, by grade twelve, both white and Negro students in the South scored lower on these tests than did white and Negro students in the North. Also, southern Negroes scored farther below southern whites than did northern Negroes below northern whites—a regional finding that correlates with the Armed Forces mental test results. (The OE study reports only regional data; by prior agreement with chief state school officers it does not reveal state-by-state test results.) The OE study also found that the average white student's achievement is less affected by the strength or weakness of his school than is that of the average Negro student.

Although there is no wholly consistent pattern, in general the study found that Negroes are offered fewer of the facilities that are most related to academic achievement (i.e., physics, chemistry, and language laboratories; libraries; textbooks; etc.). Usually greater than the majority-minority differences, however, are the regional differences.

The OE survey shows, for example, that white children generally attend elementary schools with a smaller average number of pupils in their classrooms (29) than do any of the Negroes (32). The regional breakdowns, however, show that in the Southwest the Negroes average 39 pupils per room compared to 26 per room for whites. Twice as many Negro high school students in the metropolitan Far West attend schools with language laboratories as do their counterparts in the metropolitan South (95 per cent versus 48 per cent; for whites it is 80 per cent versus 72 per cent). One hundred per cent of Negro high school students in the metropolitan Far West have access to a remedial reading teacher, compared with 46 per cent in the metropolitan South.

Over-all, Negro students are less likely to attend secondary schools that are accredited, they have less access to college preparatory curriculums, and their teachers have weaker academic credentials.

Since it is as axiomatically true in education as elsewhere that you get what you pay for, the correlation between this data, expenditure [levels by state], and the Armed Forces test results is no surprise—but neither is it very informative. It serves only as a fever gauge, saying that the patient is ill, but unable to identify his malady.

Far more precise diagnostic tools are needed to pinpoint what is happening in the nation's schools, to show what children actually learn and when and how well they learn it.

For this reason the Carnegie Corporation two years ago organized a top level committee to look into the question of whether there could or should be a national assessment of education. The committee (a private nonprofit corporation) has concluded that such an undertaking would be not only feasible, but desirable. The project has progressed from the proposal to the planning stages.

A large part of the impetus toward national assessment stems from the increasing Federal investment in education. Congress and the American taxpayer want to know what the nation is getting for its money—and not in terms of things bought but in terms of educational increments.

Twenty years ago such an assessment would have been so large an undertaking as to make it almost impossible. Today, the theory and technology of statistical sampling is so far advanced that Richard Scammon, former director of the Bureau of the Census, says a random sample of one half of one per cent of the population can provide data statistically accurate within a few percentage points.

The Carnegie committee would sample five per cent of children in the nine, thirteen, and seventeen age brackets and twenty-nine-year-old adults. The nine-year-olds represent children who are expected to have achieved the goals of primary education; the thirteen-year-olds, elementary; and the seventeen-year-olds, secondary. Adults would be surveyed for comparative purposes because they represent the major factor in determining the educational level of the nation.

No participating pupil, teacher, or school would be identified. Breakdowns would be by sex, by ethnic group, by socioeconomic level, by geographic region, and by rural, urban, and suburban residence. The committee proposes periodic assessments every three or five years.

It would be impossible to teach to the test, points out committee chairman Ralph Tyler. A teacher would be extremely unlikely to have more than one pupil tested in a five-year period, and that pupil would take only a small portion of the whole test—which is expected to require twenty hours for completion and to include seven subject areas: reading, language arts, mathematics, social studies, citizenship, fine arts, and vocational education. Prototype tests, being developed by leading educational research firms under contract to the committee, will be ready for field testing early . . . [in 1967].

Such tests, if applied nationwide, could provide a consistent and comprehensive account of the accomplishments of the nation's educational system. The general public could, for the first time, get a report of what tax dollars buy in educational achievement.

## THE WIDENING GAP IN QUALITY [2]

The present allocation of fiscal resources works against education in the central cities. The lesser resources applied to education in the cities apparently hold down educational performance, particularly in the low-income neighborhoods. Additional resources, if massive enough, would probably improve educational achievement. The political possibility of finding such resources for central city education is, at the best, uncertain.

[2] From "The Rich Get Richer & the Poor Get Poorer . . . Schools." *Carnegie Quarterly.* 14:1-3. Fall '66. Reprinted by permission.

In those dispassionate sentences, Alan K. Campbell, professor of political science and director of the metropolitan studies program at Syracuse University, sums up some of the early findings of a series of Carnegie-supported studies of large city school systems. Economists and political scientists are looking at the policies which emerge from school politics and at the ways in which the decisions which produce these policies are made—by whom, how, why and in what environments.

Professor Campbell gave some of the findings in a paper delivered last summer at Stanford University's Cubberley Conference. . . . He presented an array of facts, figures, and analyses which add up to a totally disheartening picture of the present efforts and future prospects for financing education in American cities. It is not merely that those that need it most—the city schools—are getting least. That was already known, though how badly their situation has deteriorated just recently relative to the suburbs was not known. It is the portents for the future that are alarming. For if the interested groups in the cities, including the boards of education, perform in the future as they have up to now, it appears unlikely that there will be effective voices demanding the educational resources the cities so desperately require. One may ask: "Who speaks for the city schools?"

## Plight of the Cities

As recently as 1957, annual educational expenditures per pupil in thirty-five of the largest metropolitan areas were roughly equal in the cities and their suburbs. By 1962, the suburbs were spending, on the average, $145 more per pupil than the central cities. This differential is primarily a reflection of the fact that during those years the disparity in wealth between cities and suburbs was growing.

The shocker, however, is that state aid to the schools, which one might think would be designed to redress this imbalance somewhat, discriminates *against* the cities. On the average, the suburbs receive $40 more in state aid per pupil than the cities.

Some of the Federal aid to education (which came too late to be included in the 1962 statistics) is, of course, aimed directly at disadvantaged areas. But while the Federal programs are always referred to as "massive," and while $1.25 billion per year are a lot of dollars, when they are spread over fifty states, for rural as well as city areas, the impact on any one city—or any one school —is not massive at all.

Whatever the sources of the money, local, state, or Federal, the point is that the nation is devoting many more resources to educating suburban children than city children. Or to put it another way, it is spending much more money to educate the children of the well-off than the children of the poor. And every shred of available evidence points to the conclusion that the educational needs of poor children are far greater than those of affluent children. By any measure one wants to use—pupil performance on tests, dropout rate, proportion of students going on to higher education—the output of the schools in the depressed areas of the cities is very much poorer than that of the suburbs. There is little reason to believe that even to equalize treatment would begin to close the gap. To achieve the substance rather than merely the theoretical form of equal educational opportunity requires the application of unequal resources: more rather than less to the students from poor homes.

That knowledge is, of course, what underlies the idea of compensatory education being pushed by the Federal Government and to a much lesser extent by a very few of the states. The trouble thus far with compensatory education, however, is not the idea but the few funds allocated to it. They are spread so far and so thin that only barely perceptible improvements, by and large, can be made. And barely perceptible improvements have barely perceptible effects on pupil performance.

It does little good to reduce class size from, say, 31.6 to 30.8 (like the average American family, the average American classroom seems always to contain a number of whole children plus a fraction of a child), or to raise expenditures for pupil supplies from $7.25 to $8.50, or to add one social worker to the staff of a slum high school. The evidence already in on compensatory education tends to prove this.

## Competition for Resources

There is scattered evidence, however, from the few places where it has been tried, that dramatic efforts—placing enormous concentration on the teaching of reading, for example, in very small classes—have dramatic effects. Though this evidence is not conclusive because there is not enough of it, it does suggest that some of the seemingly intractable educational problems of the cities' schools would yield before the infusion of massive resources.

The question is where to find them, or, more accurately, how to *get* them for the city schools. For the money is not hidden, after all. A great deal of it is spent in this country every day, for education and for housing, freeways, war, national parks, liquor, cosmetics, advertising, and a lot of other things. It is a question of the allocation of money, which means the establishing of priorities. That is primarily a political process, and it is heavily influenced by the clarity, vigor, and power with which spokesmen for various interests press their claims.

In education, the decision-making unit at the local level, and the principal spokesman for the schools, is the board of education. Various members of the Syracuse group are making case studies of the role of the school boards in several cities, with particular emphasis on Atlanta, Boston, Chicago, New York, and San Francisco. In the cities studied—and though there may be some striking exceptions, the rule appears to hold for most cities—the boards of education have proved to be more tax-conscious than expenditure-conscious. They have tended to tailor demands to what they calculated the tax traffic would bear rather than to hammer home the needs of the schools and the expenditure levels that would be necessary to meet them.

Since taxpayers' groups have many spokesmen and school children, especially poor ones, have few, one might have expected the boards of education to have attempted more in the way of cajoling, pleading, and demanding. This line of reasoning, however, ignores the composition of most school boards. At any rate, though boards of education might have accomplished much more if they had tried harder in the days when the cities were affluent, the question is now almost academic. Most of the big cities are strapped financially, and although some could raise more locally if they would, it is clear that the kind of money that is needed simply cannot be raised by the cities from local sources alone. Much of it will have to come from increased state and Federal aid.

### Failure of School Boards

Here the passive role of the school boards is much less easy to understand. If they despair of the possibility of getting adequate tax money at home, it is hard to fathom why they have not been leading the fight for external aid, but they have not. So far, the Campbell group concludes, the boards of education have played a relatively minor role, and "there is no evidence in the studies we have undertaken to indicate that this role is going to undergo any drastic change."

Even if it did, it is obvious that strong and active school boards alone could not bring sufficient pressure to bear on behalf of increased aid to the cities. But a coalition of school board members plus local business leaders, various civic groups, school administrators, and teachers' organizations might be able to.

"No such coalition now exists," Campbell says, though there are signs in some cities that business leaders are becoming increasingly concerned about the quality of education. As their concern grows, perhaps they will serve as rallying points for strong coalitions to speak for the cities' schools.

## WHAT'S WRONG AND RIGHT—AN OVERVIEW [3]

Robert Burns once asked—on behalf of humans in general—for the power "to see ourselves as others see us." Rarely is such a gift given but it can be therapeutic to try to seize it by standing back from one's own endeavors and imagining how another might appraise them.

[3] From "A View from Afar," by Harold Howe II, United States Commissioner of Education. *American Education*. 2:inside front cover. S. '66. *American Education* is a publication of the United States Office of Education.

If I were an educator from another planet visiting the earth and had sufficient acumen to cozen a grant from some interplanetary version of the Carnegie or Ford Foundation, here is the report I think I would file:

## Report of Earth Visit, September 1966

Around 65 per cent of Earth's inhabitants have been exposed to some form of organized education, but there is little opportunity for the remaining 35 per cent to become literate, although Earth has reasonably modern systems of communication and large unused resources which could be turned to educational purposes. In general, education is reserved for people with economic and social power. Exceptions are in the United States, Canada, and Russia, countries that try to provide education for all their citizens. Earth has not progressed to a planet-wide educational system nor has it developed a capacity for planet-wide policy planning in education.

Again in general, persons with white skin have more educational opportunity than those with black, brown, or yellow skin, although enough individuals in the latter groups succeed in advanced education to validate the assumption that skin color has nothing to do with educational capacity.

Speaking particularly of the United States, there is great similarity in educational practice, but no central system of education. The elements of similarity are too numerous to list in this report, but the following may convey a general impression of the situation:

1. Almost all children enter school at six years. No compelling reason for this practice could be discovered and a few voices advocate change. But, for the most part, these advocates merely seek to advance the age by one or two years. Few seem aware that education starts at birth and continues throughout life.

2. Each child is expected to spend the same amount of time in school as all other children. Each year students advance one grade and, in general, spend twelve years before becoming eligible

for higher education. In higher education there is a similar assumption in regard to the use of time; people typically spend four years in the lower division before moving into the upper division. Only at the graduate (or upper) division does time acquire flexibility. The result of these rigid arrangements is a great deal of what the schools call "failure." In this context, "failure" means that the student is rejected when he cannot do the work the school requires within the time allotted. There is some recognition of individual differences among pupils but most schools still require pupils to learn at a prescribed pace.

3. A great deal of time is spent away from education and the students seem to enjoy this "free" time more than time spent in school, although there are strong indications that it is seldom particularly purposeful or enjoyable. A by-product of this part-time school attendance is that the school buildings are used a small proportion of the time. (The only buildings that are used less than the schools are the churches.) In contrast, factories and other production facilities operate twenty-four hours a day. Citizens say they believe first in religious values, second in education, and only third in economic prosperity, so this pattern of facility use is, at the very least, confusing.

4. At all educational levels there is great preoccupation with what are called "standards"—a system of percentage or letter marks awarded by instructors. The standards have little to do with the individual. Instead, they appear to assume that everyone in a learning group can perform identical tasks in the same time space. The marks measure how well an individual does this. (Perhaps this is one of the reasons that students enjoy their vacations more than their education.) Small efforts to seek other approaches to describe pupil progress are detectable. For example, there are a few computer installations that build knowledge on a highly individual basis so every student can achieve success at his own rate.

### Role of "Professional Educators"

5. Teaching responsibility in the first twelve grades is held by people who call themselves "professional educators" and seem

to believe that they have a monopoly on the education of children through age eighteen. By resisting other persons interested in helping children, these professionals reject the wholesome and necessary notion that every adult should carry some responsibility for educating the young as part of his service to society.

6. The schools have a great preoccupation with what is called "attendance." (This is the habit of going to school regularly for a prescribed length of time.) Indeed, the educators seem to care more about whether the student is present than about what he is doing. In the high schools, for example, attendance is taken (i.e., the pupils are counted and accounted for) each period to make sure that no one has left school. If a student becomes interested in a book, a conversation, or an activity, he must leave it and hurry along to his next period so he will not be counted absent.

7. Students do not help plan the use of their time. At the beginning of the school year they are given a schedule which tells them where to go and what to do for the next nine months. The colleges use a unit of measurement called a "semester hour" as a basis for describing the education a person has had. This reveals how long a student has been exposed to a subject in a formal class but tells little about what he has learned. Students who learn something outside of class have no way to have their independently acquired knowledge recognized. This is also true for adults outside the formal educational structure.

8. In the United States there is no comprehensive measurement of student achievement. In fact, many professional educators oppose efforts to assess what is achieved in the schools. It is difficult to account for this in a nation which seems so interested in developing knowledge about everything else. This feeling may not be general—if the citizens were asked about periodic national assessment of educational achievement, their view might be distinctly different from that of the educators.

In spite of such criticism, it must be recognized that the United States of America has gone far beyond most Earth countries in the development of its schools. Almost all its children are involved in learning and more and more of its citizens are moving toward higher education. In addition, it does recognize that special efforts must be made for those without power or position in the society, and efforts to improve educational services for these people are being made. The United States has very recently recognized its unreasonable denial of educational opportunity for persons with dark skins and is moving to change this inequity. There is still considerable disagreement about the way to attack this problem and about the speed with which solutions should be attempted.

Because there is no central planning agency, improvements will come very slowly, but when they do come they will have the advantage of being widely accepted by all citizens.

## CATHOLIC SCHOOLS AND THEIR PROBLEMS [4]

One day, when no one was looking, it seems, the Roman Catholic school system in the United States reached giant proportions. Since 1940, the number of Catholic parochial elementary and high school students has grown from 2.4 to 5.8 million. Of all American elementary and secondary school pupils, 14 per cent attend Catholic schools, double the proportion of twenty-five years ago.

Today, then, any consideration of American education that does not take the Catholic schools into account must be found guilty of overlooking approximately every seventh student in the nation. For there are now more than six million enrolled in the nation's twelve thousand-plus Catholic educational institutions, which range from kindergartens to medical schools.

Two University of Chicago sociologists—Andrew M. Greeley, who is a Catholic priest, and Peter H. Rossi, who is not a Catholic—recently published a study of these schools, *The Education of American Catholics*. The study was financed by a grant from the Carnegie Corporation, supplemented by funds from the Office of Education of the United States Department of Health, Education, and Welfare. In an introduction, Norman M. Bradburn, acting director of the National Opinion Research Center at the . . .

[4] From "Catholics and Their Schools," by John Cogley, formerly religious news editor of The New York *Times* and now with the Center for the Study of Democratic Institutions. *Saturday Review*. 49:72-4+. O. 15, '66. Reprinted by permission.

[University of Chicago], described the book as the first systematic study of the sprawling Catholic school complex. A month after the Greeley-Rossi study appeared, another volume, *Catholic Schools in Action* . . . [ed. by R. A. Neuwien], turned up. It was also supported by a grant from the Carnegie Corporation. . . .

The two books together provide a long-overdue look into all those schools which seem to be found on every second corner in cities such as New York, Chicago, and Boston, but have somehow managed to remain as mysterious as Hindu temples to the millions of Americans who pass them every day.

Catholic school students are now found in more than 300 institutions licensed to describe themselves as centers of higher learning, and in 2,500 secondary and 10,000 elementary schools. The higher-learning sites include major universities, among them the Catholic University of America, Notre Dame, Georgetown, Fordham, St. Louis, Marquette, Boston College, and the hapless, strife-ridden St. John's of Brooklyn, which, with some 12,000 students, is the largest of all. They also include a number of good small schools, such as St. Thomas in St. Paul, Minnesota; St. Peter's in Jersey City; and Manhattan College in Riverdale, New York; as well as dozens of what Catholics themselves sometimes call "li'l ol' nuns' colleges." . . .

### A Statistical Profile

The secondary Catholic institutions are more diverse. They range from parish high schools (some with tiny enrollments, others public-school size) and the "private" low-tuition academies run by Christian Brothers, Sisters of Mercy, Franciscan Friars, or others of the Catholic teaching orders, to a few high-priced prep schools that send their graduates to Ivy League colleges. Portsmouth Priory in Rhode Island (briefly attended by Robert Kennedy) and St. Anselm's in Washington, D.C., both conducted by Benedictine monks, and the Canterbury School in Connecticut which is run by laymen (and was attended briefly by John F. Kennedy), have served as prototypes here for a few later attempts, such as the Priory schools near St. Louis, Missouri, and Woodside, California.

In the parish high schools the median tuition ranges from $76 to $100 annually. For the convent schools and boys' academies, there is a jump—between $150 . . . [and] $200 a year. Tuition costs are five times higher, though, in a few ultra-private schools such as Park Avenue's Loyola (Jesuit) and the strategically located Convents of the Sacred Heart and Marymount Schools, which are found in such places as Boca Raton, Florida; Grosse Pointe, Michigan; Lake Forest, Illinois; Upper Fifth Avenue, New York (a stretch that can boast of both a Sacred Heart and a Marymount School); and Santa Barbara, California.

Finally, there are those umpteen thousand elementary classrooms, from Maine to Hawaii. The primary schools range from two rooms in a parish auditorium set aside by a rural pastor for educational purposes, to suburban classrooms where pupils are packed as tight as cigarettes in a pack and a harassed nun is expected to handle twice the number of pupils assigned to her public-school counterpart around the corner. In between, nowadays, are the inner-city schools of the old urban parishes which are now largely attended by the minority groups who have displaced their Irish and German builders.

A few of the more fashionable convents still take grade-school children (one should not forget John-John Kennedy's alma mater, the posh St. David's on the East Side of Manhattan), but such places are exceptions to the Catholic rule. Almost all Catholic elementary schools in America are parish-connected.

In all, the Catholic schools employ 200,000 teachers. About two thirds of this division in the church militant are priests, seminarians, brothers, and nuns, content to work for subsistence pay. In most parishes, in addition to these minimal salaries, the pastor is expected to maintain the convent where the nun-teachers live.

Motherhouses, as the major convents of the various sisterhoods are called, receive a certain percentage of the meager income their members earn. This money is necessary for the administrative overhead of the order, the education of young sisters, and the care of sick and retired members. Where parishes are very poor, however, the parochial schools are sometimes subsidized by the orders that conduct them.

About 65,000 parochial school teachers are laymen. They are almost always underpaid, are generally underprivileged, and are frequently underprepared for their jobs. In all but a very few places they, too, receive salaries far below the educational sea-level. The median pay is less than $4,000 annually—$2,000 below public school standards.

Lay teachers are not vowed to poverty. Not surprisingly, then, they are rarely content to receive so little. Their chief complaint, however, is not the low pay they get but the abiding sense they have of not being accepted by their clerical colleagues as professional peers. This complaint is heard in university and grade school alike. In many parochial schools, the Notre Dame investigators found, there are even two kinds of faculty meetings. One, open to all teachers, deals with routine administrative and disciplinary matters; the other, confined to members of the order that conducts the school, deals with questions of academic substance and the establishment of basic educational standards.

Many lay teachers who know that they were pressed into service only because of a shortage of qualified clergy or nuns begin idealistically, but soon end their service to the Catholic school system with a bitter sense of second-class ecclesiastical citizenship. It should also be acknowledged, however, that especially at the primary level the laymen are frequently second-class teachers lacking professional training. In a parish I know well, for example, a lady parishioner who had originally been hired to drive the school bus suddenly found herself presiding over a classroom because she was the only person available for the job. The same sort of thing has undoubtedly happened elsewhere, especially since Mothers Superior these days, stung by widespread public criticism of Catholic education, are reluctant about sending their nuns out to teach before they have been professionally qualified. Educational standards for young teaching sisters have leaped enormously in recent years.

Pastors, in competition with the public school system, do not have a wide choice from which to pick the ever-increasing number of lay teachers they need. The Notre Dame study shows that there is extraordinary unevenness in teacher preparation throughout the system. Of the elementary teachers, lay and religious, about half have earned a bachelor's degree. In the nation's public schools, in contrast, the figure runs as high as 98 per cent and as low as 28 per cent. About three fourths of the Catholic high school teachers are college graduates. In the public high schools, virtually all teachers have a degree.

The Catholic schools, it is always important to note, are almost wholly supported by private means, but are expected by their clients to maintain standards set by publicly supported schools. Father Greeley and Dr. Rossi made the point that "of all modernized countries, the United States is the only one which maintains an extensive denominational school system financed by nongovernmental sources."

Only a handful of the schools benefit from endowments. About half the elementary and 77 per cent of the secondary institutions survive on direct tuition charges. However, tuition ($25 or less is the annual median for the elementary school, with an equal amount of yearly "charges") usually needs to be generously supplemented by parish funds. In a few dioceses there are no tuition charges at all, school costs are met directly by the parish. (Contributions given to a church, it might be noted, are tax-exempt, though tuition payments to a religious school are not.)

Support from the various dioceses is not anywhere near as high as might be expected by those who think of the Roman Catholic Church as the most centralized institution of all. The Notre Dame study states that only thirty-four high schools in the United States get more than half their income from a bishop's office.

Merely to keep up with population growth, according to the Notre Dame projection, Catholic schools will, by 1968-69, have to take in a million more students than the number registered in 1962-63—or more people than can be found in any one of seventeen states in the Union. To hold the present line, 21,000 additional religious teachers and 10,500 lay teachers will be required. Additional school construction alone will cost more than $721 million. Even if all these miracles are accomplished, the schools will still be educating fewer than half the pupils in the United States baptized as Catholics. Even now, the schools can find no room for about one fifth of those who apply. Many more would apply if parents thought their children had a chance to get in. The percentage of those turned down does not promise to shrink as the number of children grows and the number of teaching sisters diminishes.

The process of selecting who get the desired places in the Catholic classroom varies from place to place. Almost everywhere parents must be members in good standing of the parish. Where applicants exceed the number the school can accommodate, which is almost everywhere, admission is based on the length of time in the parish, the amount of church activity the family engages in, and on whether parents use the "envelope" in making contributions. (Without the envelope, there is no way of knowing who contributed how much or how often.) As the Greeley-Rossi study points out, the schools make the elite more elite.

How good are these schools? They should be judged, it seems, by two sets of criteria; first, the ordinary academic standards applied to educational systems, and second, the particular standards which schools with the special purpose of carrying on religious education and developing religious understanding have set for themselves. In addition, there are questions about the education offered. For example: Does the religious separatism of parochial education strengthen prejudiced habits of thought and encourage stereotypes about persons of races, nationalities, and religions not found in the schools? Are Catholic school graduates trained largely by monastics prepared to hold their own in the very secular world where they will have to earn a living?

Together, the Greeley-Rossi and Notre Dame studies throw light on such questions.

## Some Advantages and Shortcomings

How good are Catholic schools simply as schools? How do they compare with public schools?

Before answering the questions, the shortcomings and advantages should be noted. The Catholic schools are almost scandalously overcrowded, though there has been a notable improvement on this score in recent years. Their teachers have less academic preparation. Finally, they operate on a much lower budget. Even though the merely nominal pay of the sisters makes up for some of the difference, it is not enough to balance the amount spent on each child.

On the advantageous side, it must be kept in mind that the Church schools can pick and choose their students. Unruly and undisciplined pupils often end up in the public schools because the nuns are in a position to demand a certain standard of behavior. From many teachers' point of view, this is an enormous benefit.

With all this duly noted, it must then be recorded that on the basis of comparative records, students in Catholic schools are "superior," both in academic achievement and in learning potential. This really should not surprise anyone. The Notre Dame authors, for example, modestly point out that the superiority they found can be attributed largely to the "relatively selective" admissions policies of the schools. There is no note in their report of what a critical bishop at the Vatican Council called "Catholic triumphalism."

The parochial schools, however, are not all *that* selective, and the overcrowding and heavy teaching loads and limited budgets with which they operate might have suggested that they would be significantly less advanced. Over the years, vague charges of academic inferiority have been hurled against the nun-directed schools and have frequently been taken as the gospel truth, so to speak, by persons who could not imagine why they shouldn't be true. It seems only fair, now that evidence of massive testing is available, to acknowledge that, if anything, children in Catholic schools are academically privileged.

Thousands of elementary school pupils were given the Stanford Achievement Test and two mental ability measures, the Kuhlman-Anderson Test and Otis Mental Ability Test, for the Notre Dame report. High-school students were given the Metropolitan Achievement Test, High School Battery and Otis Mental Ability Test. The results were these: IQ's of elementary pupils averaged out to 110, a sign of superior academic learning potential. Eighty-four per cent had achievement scores at or above the national norms. There were similar findings for high school students. About 17 per cent exceeded the national norms in academic achievement; more than 80 per cent were classified as reaching "total potential" in language arts, social studies, mathematics, and science.

The Greeley-Rossi study concentrated on the relationship between Catholic education and adult religious behavior. The authors found that the link between the religious education offered in a Catholic school and adult behavior is notably stronger in those who were brought up in devout families. In other words, classroom religious education is much more likely to "take" if it is bolstered by the example of parents.

### Effect of Religious Education

Other Greeley-Rossi findings are these:

Males who attended Catholic colleges are notably more religiously observant than Catholics who stopped their religious education before reaching college. The difference here turned out to be so great that the authors concluded that "religious education will probably produce the effect its supporters seek for it only when it is 'comprehensive' (from first grade to college degree)."

Present-day high school students show a much stronger correlation between religious education and religious behavior than their older brothers and sisters. This could be the result of an improvement in religious educational techniques, or it could be because religious fidelity tends to erode after graduation. The authors say they were led to believe, however, that where Catholic education was not strengthened at home, its effects were short-ranged; where school and family work together, the impact on the young is a lasting phenomenon.

The Notre Dame investigators devised their own test to measure the understanding of the Catholic religion gained by parochial school pupils. They decided that, on the whole, the students did well. Girls in all-girl schools, they found, showed the best understanding of Catholicism—or at least they provided the most "advanced" answers to the questions asked.

The Notre Dame test was designed to measure "advanced," "moderate," "moralistic," "conventional" and "nominalistic" religious comprehensions. A typical question was the following:

The chief value of the life, sufferings, and death of Our Lord (Jesus) is that He thereby:
   a) earned for us God's grace and everlasting life [advanced]
   b) showed His unlimited love for us [moderate]
   c) taught us how to live, suffer, and die [moralistic]
   d) set us free from sin and sin's penalty [conventional]
   e) proved to doubters that He was a real man [nominalistic]

A total of 56 per cent of those queried selected the highly desired "advanced" or "moderate" responses, 32 per cent chose the "conventional," and only 12 per cent the "moralistic" or "nominalistic."

Father Greeley and Dr. Rossi, who gave considerable attention to the matter, found no evidence that Catholic schools were "divisive." Community involvement, concern about "worldly problems," and attitudes toward other groups were not significantly affected, they decided, by attendance at Church schools.

The majority of Catholic-school students said their three best friends were also Catholics, but this reply turned out to be no different than the answer given to that question by Catholics in public schools. The same was true for Protestants and Jews. "Americans apparently choose their friends from their own religious group, no matter what kind of education they have," the authors concluded.

Greeley and Rossi also found that Catholic collegians are more "liberal" than Catholics who do not attend Catholic colleges and, where anti-Semitism is concerned, considerably more "liberal" than college-educated Protestants—a conclusion also sustained by the recent Glock-Stark studies sponsored by B'nai B'rith. The Notre Dame investigators found, however, that only 47 per cent of the students surveyed gave an unbiased response to this statement: "There is something strange and different about Jews. It is hard to know what they are thinking or planning, or what makes them tick." Less bias was shown in response to a similar stereotyping of Negroes. But no more than two thirds to three fourths of the students were ever on the side of the angels when tests of bias were made. The Notre Dame investigators concluded from this that though the Catholic schools may not be doing any worse than others in combating prejudice, they are not doing well enough.

## What Future for Catholic Schools?

Catholic school graduates, Greeley and Rossi found, do slightly better in achieving success in professional life than do Catholics who attended other schools. As a possible explanation they point out that students in a Catholic school do not occupy the minority status they might have in a public institution and that their self-confidence is therefore strengthened at a crucial time in life. Later, they found, the Catholic school graduate seems to adapt as readily to the religiously mixed world of business and the professions as anyone else and manifests neither more nor less clannishness than his fellow Catholics.

Are Catholic schools, then, still necessary? The question is asked by some who feel that anything that pulls Catholics away from others is bad for the Church as well as for the nation. It is asked by others who feel that the home and the parish church, rather than the school, are the proper places for religious education. It is asked by some who believe that the idea of a "Catholic culture," which was supposed to be transmitted by the Church's schools, is an anachronism and that the work of contemporary Christians is to wrestle with the problems common to all men and express their religious concerns in a "secular" mode.

Others question in dollars-and-cents terms the feasibility of continuing the Catholic school system. They point out the rising cost of education. An even greater inequality in physical resources enjoyed by the parochial and the public schools will be brought about by Federal aid to public schools. There is also the sheer financial burden parents feel in maintaining a separate system in addition to paying full taxes for schools and other services their children do not use. When the Catholic population was largely composed of urban renters, the cost of maintaining two systems was not as evident as it is today for the home-owning Catholic suburbanite, who is very much aware of school taxes and the benefits he is losing because his children are in a parochial school.

Father Greeley and Dr. Rossi concluded that maintaining the schools was not necessary for the survival of American Catholicism. They found, for example, that of all Catholics who attended public schools and whose parents attended public schools, three of every five attend Mass weekly. If the schools were to be closed tomorrow, the University of Chicago authors imply, there would be no mass apostasy; the Church would probably have just as many adherents in the next generation as it has now.

However, Greeley and Rossi do not expect the schools to be closed down tomorrow, or the day after tomorrow, or the day after that; nor do they expect them to be "phased out." They write: "A system which involves one out of every seven school children in our republic does not go out of business, either all at once or gradually." Being for or against such a system, they say, is like being for or against the Rocky Mountains—it might be great fun but it does not alter reality.

## II. THE FORCES OF REFORM

### EDITOR'S INTRODUCTION

It would appear that pressures for reform in the schools work from two directions: from the top of society down and from the bottom of society up. At the top the nation's industrial managers, experts, and technicians are voracious in their demands for more quality in greater quantities—for vast reserves of "brainpower" to man the country's industrial, commercial and scientific establishments. At the bottom are the poor and the culturally deprived. Today, as never before, they are organizing to demand that the syndrome of poverty and poor schools that has entrapped them will be broken for the benefit of their children. When the history of education in this century is written, in fact, the role of the civil rights movement in reform may well bulk large.

In any case, pressures from both directions are prompting changes in our schools. A host of special programs are being established both for the gifted youngster and for the culturally deprived. The pressures, in fact, have generated counterpressures in the form of complaints by some educators that the average student, neither gifted nor deprived, is becoming "the forgotten youth in today's America."

This section explores in detail some of the forces of reform now making their influence felt in the schools. In the first article the "search for brainpower" is discussed by the editor of the Columbia College alumni magazine, who raises this intriguing question: In a democracy in which equal treatment of all students is a cherished ideal, how can the specially gifted youngster be developed to his full potential? The second article deals with the failure of vocational education in America. Although some 80 per cent of all high school students fail to go on to college and find college preparatory curricula unsuited to their needs, vocational education remains the neglected step-child of our education establishment.

In the third article a professor of social relations at Johns Hopkins University makes the startling revelation, backed by an extensive survey, that children of minority groups have a more serious educational deficiency at the end of their schooling than they did at the start—that, in other words, disadvantaged children actually emerge from our educational establishments relatively less well off than when they entered. In the final article, the editors of *U.S. News & World Report* raise some questions about the attention being showered upon both gifted and disadvantaged children and ask whether the average youngster is not suffering from neglect as a result.

## THE SEARCH FOR "BRAINPOWER" [1]

In the unpromising year of 1930, President Herbert Hoover called a White House Conference on Child Health and Protection, the purpose of which was to discuss "for the first time in history" what it called "special education"—classes, schools, and teachers for those who were not ordinary children. Its list of special groups included the blind, the crippled, the deaf, those with speech problems, the mentally retarded, those with health problems (heart trouble, malnutrition, tuberculosis, epilepsy), those with behavior problems (emotionally disturbed and chronic delinquents), and—last on the agenda—gifted children.

Thirty-five years later, in 1964, President Lyndon Johnson established a Presidential Scholars Program for gifted high school youths to recognize, as he put it, "the most precious resource of the United States—the brainpower of its young people." The National Merit Corporation, the National Science Foundation, various state governments, many municipal and suburban school systems, and numerous other agencies now currently display intense interest in cultivating the academically top-notch. Publicists shout about the desperate shortage in the "national supply" of scientists and other intellectuals. To talk about gifted young-

[1] From article by George C. Keller, editor of *Columbia College Today*, the Columbia College alumni magazine. *Public Interest.* no 4:59-69. Summer '66. Reprinted by permission.

sters as if they were simply a special problem group, like the deaf or the emotionally disturbed, is today almost unthinkable.

Obviously, there has been a remarkable change in the United States during the past thirty-five years in our thinking about the use and the place of intellect in society. But if intellect has suddenly become a major national asset, just what do we know today about identifying and developing "brainpower"?

## From Terman to World War II

In his revealing semiautobiographical Bingham lecture at Berkeley, Lewis Madison Terman, the Stanford psychologist who pioneered in the study of the gifted, remarked that the prevailing attitude, while he was a graduate student at Clark University, was "early ripe, early rot." He recounts how he began his great study of 1,000 gifted youngsters in 1921 to test the validity of this attitude—"to find out what traits characterize children of high IQ and . . . to see what kind of adults they become." To the astonishment of the American educational world, and even to his own mild surprise, the first results of Terman's study in 1925 disclosed that the intellectually gifted, for the most part, were far above average in vigor, readiness to work hard, and appreciation of school, slightly above average in health, conduct, and emotional maturity, and not below average in physical skills. They were not oddballs, but fairly normal youngsters. Moreover, as Terman followed his gifted youths through the years, they became, to an amazing degree (70 per cent), men who graduated from college and who went on to occupy positions of authority and distinction in society; very few turned out to be "maladjusted." Terman's findings, supported by the work of such men as Columbia's Edward Thorndike, Ohio State's Sidney Pressey, and Leta Hollingworth, were shattering to leading educators, most of whom had unconsciously absorbed the prevailing bourgeois-philistine notion of gifted children.

Earlier, there had been little interest in identifying and nourishing the academically gifted students in the primary and secondary schools. The first recorded experiment with especially able youngsters was the adoption in St. Louis, in 1868, of the "flexible promotion scheme," or "skipping," as it came to be known. In 1918 the National Education Association issued a remarkable report, *The Cardinal Principles of Secondary Education.* It argued that curricula need not be fixed but could be multi-purpose; that is, special sections of classes or "enriched" courses could be set up for the more talented, instead of "skipping" them out of school at an earlier age. The suggestion was picked up in some places; by 1928, forty cities in twenty-three states had classes for gifted children—with a grand total of four thousand pupils in them.

But the objections to separating the gifted were loud and many. The schools at the time were thought to have three main purposes: to train for business and the professions, to provide a base for political democracy, and to serve as a social melting pot for persons of different national origins, religions, and—in the North and West—different skin colors. Special sections or enriched courses for some pupils seemed to serve none of these purposes. On the contrary, it was felt that businessmen and professionals might become more conceited and snobbish and would develop dangerously unbalanced views of life because of a lack of intimacy with average and below-average people in their youth. Democracy, too, would suffer as a result of such "elitism;" and the "Americanization" process would be hurt because many of the natural leaders of the "melting" operation would be absent.

In the 1930's the objectors to special classes, aided by the shortage of money for educational purposes, had their way. There was a widespread abandonment of the relatively few special sections that were in operation, and the mixed classroom—with extra homework for the mentally quick—became the favored pattern. Small special classes, additional aids, and extra efforts were widely established—to help the *least* academically talented and the other problem youngsters to which the Hoover Conference gave attention. In 1940 there were 604 cities in the United States giving special attention to the mentally deficient, but only 36 cities in 1950 reported any special attention to the mentally extraordinary.

## A Sudden Passion for Intellect

The advent of World War II, with its need for experts, changed that order of priorities slightly, but not as much as might be expected. Five years after the war ended, the place of the gifted in the schools was not substantially different from what it had been in 1928.

But in the 1950's there was another startling reversal of social priorities. The nation "discovered" the value of intellect, or "brainpower," as it came to be called. In 1950 the Educational Policies Commission of the NEA issued a statement on the Education of the Gifted; in 1951 the National Science Foundation was set up, and the Ford Foundation started a program to get very bright sixteen-year-olds into college a year earlier; in 1953 the National Manpower Council deplored "the acute shortages among highly skilled professional, scientific, and technical workers needed in defense and essential civilian activities," and the Advanced Placement Program was begun; and in 1954 Dael Wolfe's influential *America's Resources of Specialized Talent,* sponsored by the Commission on Human Resources, studied the "potential supply" of intellect for the polity.

While Federal Government officials, confronted with the exigencies of a continuing Cold War, hastened to increase the supply of brainpower, the challenges of an increasingly technical and intricately organized economy forced businessmen and economists to restudy their view of the place and value of highly talented individuals in economic growth. Although some political economists from Adam Smith to John Stuart Mill and Alfred Marshall had argued the importance of talented persons to a nation's prosperity, most economists—both capitalist and Marxist—have focused, and still focus, their attention on the relation among *things,* on goods, monies, services. In the late 1950's, a new school of young economists—John Vaizey in England, Gino Martinoli in Italy, Odd Aukrust in Norway, Columbia University's Gary Becker and Chicago's Theodore Schultz in the United States—began to argue that economics makes little sense unless one includes *human capital,* and that economic growth for developed countries and development for poor countries depend chiefly upon that resource, particularly in an industrial-scientific age. . . .

As a result of this and similar attitudes, the United States has increased its investment in schools, colleges, universities, and their personnel from 4 per cent of the total "physical capital" in 1900 to over 30 per cent in 1965. In 1955, businessmen who had, thirty years ago, scoffed at any attention paid to the gifted, set up the National Merit Corporation to ferret out the nation's most academically talented secondary school students and to assure that each of them had the opportunity of a college education. . . .

### Who Is Academically Gifted?

Who is an "academically talented" youngster? According to the 1931 Hoover Conference report, "it has been practically agreed that 120 IQ may be safely taken as the lower limit" although "some systems do not go below 130 IQ." The National Education Association, or NEA, which tends to be very egalitarian —"No one group of students, including the academically talented, must gain educational advantages at the expense of any other group" (1959)—used for its Academically Talented Project students with IQ above 116, or one standard deviation above the national mean of 100. Frank Copley, in *The American High School and the Talented Student,* wrote: "For this report I should say that academic talent begins at about IQ 120 or 125, or in terms of the College Board's . . . [Scholastic Aptitude Tests], at a score of 600 or 620, both verbal and quantitative." Several states use 130 IQ as a demarcation point for the gifted, and that is where Leta Hollingworth drew the line, although Lewis Terman preferred to make 140 IQ the measure of a gifted person. One study disclosed that the highest achievers in the *Dictionary of American Biography* are mostly 130 IQ or above; relatively few are as low as, or lower than, 120 IQ. Of those in the top fifth of their secondary school classes, Dael Wolfe found, 92 per cent with 130 IQ or above graduated from college, but after that the percentage drops off sharply, indicating that perhaps 130 IQ might be a meaningful cutoff point. (The average IQ of Ph.D. recipients in the United States is 130.)

The most recent description, now used by most Federal education officials, gives three levels of academic superiority.

1. The academically talented, or those with 116 IQ (Binet), one standard deviation above the mean of normal distribution. This group constitutes about 20 per cent of the total school population, and may be as high as 60 per cent of the students in better private schools or schools in a high socioeconomic community. The College Board scores of this group are usually 450 or above in both the verbal and mathematics areas. Students in this category can graduate from an average college, and some are able to do graduate work at the less demanding universities. (Most of the creatively talented, many of the psychosocially talented, and a good portion of the kinesthetically talented are in this category, at the least.)

2. The gifted, or those with 132 IQ, two standard deviations above the mean. This group comprises about 3 per cent of the school population. Their College Board SAT's are usually both above 600. They can graduate from any college in the nation and many of them can earn professional degrees and Ph.D.'s at any university.

3. The highly gifted, or those with 148 IQ, three standard deviations above the mean. Only .1 per cent of all the young are found in this category. They usually achieve College Board scores of 725 in the verbal and mathematics SAT's. Their potential is unlimited.

Using 1964-65 school enrollment figures, the percentage of secondary school students in each category looks like this: of 12.8 million secondary school students, 2.56 million were academically talented, 384,000 were gifted, 12,800 were highly gifted.

To look at it another way: of the approximately 2.3 million secondary school graduates in June, 1965, roughly 550,000 were academically talented, 90,000 were gifted, and 3,000 were highly gifted. Nevertheless, around 1.3 million graduates—more than twice the number of academically talented in the Class of '65—

enrolled at colleges and universities in the fall of 1965. It is not surprising that something like 20 per cent drop out of college during, or at the end of, the freshman year, and only 45 per cent are graduated from college.

## What Makes Them Gifted?

The academically talented or gifted persons are not only statistics, however; they are products of particular circumstances. It may be extremely difficult to identify the truly extraordinary students, and hard to classify them, but we have fairly good information on the characteristics of intellectually superior children, and increasingly better knowledge about their formation.

Academically gifted youngsters tend to come from small families (they are frequently first children), from well-educated and productive homes (Terman found that 30 per cent of the children of gifted people are also gifted), from high socioeconomic backgrounds (each year 40 per cent of the National Merit Scholars are discovered to need no scholarship to even the most expensive colleges), from certain ethnic-cultural origins (English, German, and Jewish families are more productive of intellectual children than Italian, Negro, or Polish families), and from particular religions (Jews produce more intellectuals than Protestants, who produce more than Catholics).

One highly important fact is that there is mounting evidence that the primary determinant in developing gifted children is the family. Considering that most persons concerned about raising the intellectual level of Americans concentrate on improving the schools, this may well be the most significant oversight in American education. . . .

A money-minded nation like the United States is inclined to overlook family influence and regard poverty as the sole cause of low academic achievement. Similarly, the American optimistic view of human nature, the desire to play down religious differences, the change from a Puritan ethic to a "fun" ethic, and the swelling disdain for leaders and authority also cause many in the country to ignore the important role of child discipline and training, family religiocultural attitudes, hard work, and parental encouragement. It is much easier to blame bureaucratic bungling, or the poor schools, for a student's failure. To be sure, both the schools and their officials are far from what they should be. But the vital influence of family cannot be neglected—particularly when more and more learning and value formation goes on outside the schools, through the mass media, advertising, and social activities.

Two examples of the predominant influence of the family, despite adverse socioeconomic circumstances, can suffice here. One is what Samuel Stouffer calls "the amazing success story of the American Jew," who, despite being poor, produced many individuals of high academic achievement. The other is something that was caught by John Anderson: "Terman pointed out that there were seven times as many children with high IQ's within families of the professional class as in the class of unskilled laborers. But since the class of unskilled laborers at that time was ten times as large as the professional class, actually there were, in absolute numbers, more gifted children in the United States within the laboring group than within the professional group." Poverty is obviously a strong deterrent to learning; but children from certain kinds of families learn despite its stultifying effects —while others don't.

### What Can the Schools Do?

But it is not easy to know what to do about families, whereas we do have some ideas of what to do about schooling. It has now been fairly conclusively demonstrated, for instance, that young children can tackle much more mathematics and science— and enjoy it—than anyone dreamed fifteen years ago. It is stifling and backward, in this increasingly scientific-technical age, to ask a boy or girl to wait, say, until his junior year in secondary school, when he or she is sixteen, to begin chemistry, especially since gifted mathematicians and scientists seemingly blossom young or not at all. Also, foreign languages should be taught better, earlier, and more broadly, given America's increasingly international involvement. As late as 1957, 56 per cent of the public high schools in the United States did not offer *any* foreign language.

There is some information coming in that may be of great help in nurturing more gifted students. Benjamin Bloom and a few others have argued—not entirely convincingly—that over one half of a person's intellectual capacity is developed by the time he is four years old. (The importance of the family again!) This has led to a sudden and entirely welcome enthusiasm for nursery schools and prenursery programs, especially in areas where there are many poor people. Another study has shown that gifted children associate cheerfully with most other children in their classes until the fourth or fifth grade, when they begin to develop a sharp awareness of themselves and form friendships mainly among other bright children. Is the fifth grade the place to begin special sections or enriched courses? Also, gifted children are often more popular than others in the class until the eighth or ninth grade, when peer group values become dominant and the gifted are pressured to conform. Isn't high school, therefore, a place to intensify the awards and recognition for the gifted, or to consider special schools for them?

Other information also suggests the need for major reassessments. Henry Chauncey, president of Educational Testing Service, said recently: "You can predict how well an individual will do in college just about as accurately at age fourteen as at age eighteen. This to most people is a rather surprising fact. . . . [But] the growth of intellectual abilities, as reflected by standardized test scores, has stabilized by this age period." Shouldn't we do more testing at ages thirteen and fourteen, and less at sixteen and seventeen? And shouldn't we drastically improve the quality of primary . . . and junior high school teachers?

John Flanagan, reporting on the results of the United States Office of Education's Project Talent in 1964, found that, "20 to 30 per cent of the students in grade 9 know more about many subject-matter fields than does the average student in grade 12. Variability within grades is greater than variability between grades." Doesn't this argue for more, not less, reordering of secondary school instruction? (Probably 80 per cent of the country's high schools still have no systematic program for encouraging gifted students!)

Information of this kind hints that the United States should be moving toward a 4-4-4 system of education, with a lower, middle, and high school. The lower school might remain small and a neighborhood school with a mixture of academic talents— comprehensive schools in the old sense—with extra homework for the academically talented, special projects for the gifted, and tutoring and counseling for the below average. (IQ and other academic tests are least reliable for the early years.) The middle school, grades 5 to 8, could draw children from a wider area and have two "tracks," a fast and a slow one, with children in the academically talented (116 IQ or above) category in the fast section. The high school might be sectional (in metropolises), city-wide, or regional, no smaller than one thousand students, as many already are; and it could be "multi-tracked" in each course, or, in large cities, somewhat specialized by student interests and talents, e.g., science, music, art, social studies, etc.

As for the very gifted, those with 148 IQ or above, it would appear that they should receive individual attention at all levels, and be accelerated in most cases. All good colleges should entertain early admission—a year or two ahead of time—for these rare youths.

## The Task of Reconciliation

American education in the past few years has entered a tortuously difficult period, as the schools and colleges have been asked to solve more and more of the community's and society's problems. In particular, they have been given two new huge and urgent tasks: that of identifying and developing the gifted student —fast—and that of helping to eliminate Negro scholastic inferiority—quickly. The two tasks, intellectual excellence and equality, requiring the schools to move in different directions, are tearing many schools in half. Zealots like to attribute the tensions exclusively to bigotry, selfishness, or anti-intellectualism, and they may be sometimes right in part; but there are legitimate national issues behind the local struggles.

Obviously, a complex, highly technological society faced with serious international problems requires ever greater numbers of persons with developed intellects. The United States faces a scarcity of academic talent, as numerous studies have shown; and the argument for better nurturing of the gifted, through distinctive courses, separate sections, and even special schools, is a powerful one.

Yet, the need to achieve a fully democratic and egalitarian society seems equally imperative, both on humanitarian and internationally political grounds. Such efforts as the recent drive by many Negroes and some of their white supporters to abolish New York's special schools because they are "undemocratic" and detrimental to a more integrated school system are entirely understandable, too. There may be a very real danger of leveling, in the worst sense, in the one position; but there may also be a genuine danger of erecting a meritocracy—a twentieth century form of enlightened despotism—in the other.

Neither "equal treatment" in the schools nor "equality of opportunity" in the schools is a discardable ideal. Unfortunately, it is easier to celebrate them in the abstract than to reconcile them in practice. There is an inherent tension between equality and excellence—though not, one hopes, a contradiction. How the school systems cope with this tension is perhaps the fundamental issue in educational policy in our lifetime, as well as one of the key determinants of the future social arrangements of American society.


## THE WASTE OF MANPOWER [2]

The biggest failure of American education is not its inability to produce more scientists than Russia. It is the way in which it is turning millions of young people into unemployables. This

[2] From "Learning to Be Unemployable," by Edward T. Chase, a consultant and writer on public affairs. *Harper's Magazine.* 226:33-40. Ap. '63. Copyright © 1963 by Harper's Magazine, Inc. Reprinted from the April, 1963 issue of *Harper's Magazine* by permission of the author.

fact is as little understood as it is shocking. Because of it, job-hunting youths face a grimmer prospect in the 1960's than their elders did in 1933 at the depth of the Great Depression, when the unemployment figure stood at a record 24.9 per cent.

Already today, in many cities, unemployment among youths equals—and is often double or triple—this Depression rate. And the outlook is worsening. In the closing days of 1962, while general unemployment remained at a fixed level, the number of young people out of work leaped upward by 100,000. And another 100,000 increase was recorded in the first figures on unemployment for 1963. [While over-all unemployment has fallen somewhat from its 1962-63 levels, high unemployment among youth remains a major national problem.—Ed.]

This menacing situation is a direct consequence of the gross imbalance in our educational system. Its attention has been overwhelmingly concentrated on the 20 per cent of students who go through college. The vocational future of the other 80 per cent has been either ignored or sabotaged by an archaic system of job training. It is a system that produces unneeded farmers, cabinet-makers, and weavers, while the demand is rising for business-machine repairmen, chefs, auto mechanics, and electrical service-men—to mention only a few of the skills in short supply.

A self-serving lobby of vocational educationists perpetuates this training in moribund trades; at the same time it has intensified the youth unemployment crisis by tightening the standards of admission to vocational schools. In the academic high schools, on the other hand, there is, in the main, not even the semblance of preparation for work. Ninety per cent of all U.S. schools offer no training for jobs in industry; 95 per cent offer none in selling or merchandising although there are now more job opportunities in these fields than in production; only about 18 per cent of high school students in urban areas are getting any sort of preparation for work. Indeed the Federal Government spends ten times as much on the National School Lunch Program as on vocational education—which commands only 4 per cent of all current expenditures on public education. [With the subsequent introduction of such Federal programs as the Job Corps, this percentage has of course risen.—Ed.]

## A National Scandal

For years this national scandal has been swept under the rug. There is, however, now some hope that the shortcomings of our job-training efforts will be aired—and even that steps will be taken to remedy them. For our archaic vocational education system has suddenly become the vital tool in a massive national effort to train unemployed people for new jobs under the Manpower Development and Training Act passed by Congress at the . . . [1962] session. It is in our long-ignored vocational schools— in afternoon and evening classes—that men and women who may have been out of work for months will, it is hoped, be taught trades that will make them self-supporting. Large sums of Federal money will be poured into this program. And in the process local school boards, employers, and many other Americans who have never worried about what went on inside vocational schools will be brought face to face with their inadequacy. . . .

The need to halt this wasteful neglect becomes increasingly urgent as the demand for unskilled workers continues to shrink. Unskilled jobs today account for only 5 per cent of all U.S. employment. In the 1960's on the average some 2.5 million jobs will be eliminated annually by automation. Most dismaying is the yearly loss of a quarter of a million "entry" jobs, the kind whereby youth matriculate into the work world. Simultaneously there will be a spectacular explosion of young men and women from fourteen to twenty-five years old into the labor force—50 per cent more of them than in the 1950's. But few of them will find work unless we take emergency steps to prepare them for the kind of jobs that will need doing. Difficult though this may seem, it is by no means impossible, for a good deal of precise information is available as to the technological and occupational changes that lie ahead.

Projections provided by the Division of Manpower and Employment Statistics of the U.S. Department of Labor show, for instance, that we will need 50,000 new carpenters annually in the 1960's, 5,000 new tool- and diemakers and appliance servicemen, and 10,000 new plumbers. We will also need many times the current supply of technicians—aids to engineers, guards, dry cleaners, policemen, and waiters. We will need more stenographers and secretaries but fewer typists (more copying will be done by duplicating machines). Similarly there will be a decline —due to technological and social changes—in the demand for refrigerator mechanics, lithographers, machinists, cashiers, paperhangers, and telephone linemen.

Projections like these should, one would think, be a matter of vital concern to the people who run our vocational education system. But if you visit almost any vocational school, you will find its program incredibly irrelevant to the facts of work in the 1960's. To understand why this is so, one must pause for a brief look at the little-known history of vocational education—or "vo-ed" as it is known in the shorthand of the educationists.

Keystone of our vocational education system—unaltered to this day though other laws have supplemented it—is the Smith-Hughes Act, which Woodrow Wilson signed in 1917. At that time, about a third of all American workers were farmers and the accent was heavily on training for agriculture. It still is— even though only one eighteenth of our labor force now works on the farm (and often not in full-time jobs). . . . [In 1963] as in 1917, nearly half of the annual $7 million of Federal money provided under this basic legislation (it is given to the states in perpetuity on a dollar-for-dollar basis) goes to farm training. This law and its supplements are very precise about just what this means. States cannot be reimbursed for training in such things as food processing, marketing, maintenance of farm machinery, or irrigation—all fields that now employ more rural people than actual farming does.

Across the country a third of all vocational education funds— Federal, state, and local combined—are still spent on training farmers, although at present only one young applicant in ten can hope to find a job on a farm when he leaves school. Even

New York City is the beneficiary—if that's the word—of farm-teaching funds. The city maintains and is expanding a farm school in Flushing, a semisuburban area half an hour by subway from Times Square. . . .

Under the Smith-Hughes Act, while nearly one half of the annual Federal grant goes into teaching Adam to delve (or its equivalent), 20 per cent is allocated to teaching Eve to spin. To be sure, home economics has progressed a bit beyond spinning and weaving. But most of the courses consist of disorganized, mediocre instruction in skills that have little relevance to the age of supermarkets.

Dr. Chester E. Swanson, Director of the Presidential Panel, when I talked to him in Washington not long ago, called the present stress on home economics absurd. Most enlightened educators agree with him. Yet for years home economics has enrolled the largest number of students in the federally reimbursed vocational education program. Indeed, some home economists are now urging that boys too should devote part of the school day to "the homemaking arts." Admiral Rickover should really have a talk with these ladies.

## Hardy Though Moribund

Vo-ed, as it is practiced today, is not only fantastically biased in favor of farming and home economics. It also teaches skills and uses equipment which are often hopelessly obsolete—even in such categories as trade and industrial education. Dr. Swanson recalled, for instance, that in the 1940's when he became a school official in Allentown, Pennsylvania, cabinetmaking was the rage. On investigating he discovered there had been no jobs for cabinetmakers in Allentown for years. However, teachers of this trade had tenure and expensive equipment. He was up against a stone wall when he tried to reduce the staff and beef up more pertinent parts of the vo-ed curriculum.

In addition, Federal money goes to training in certain specified occupations. The broadest category is trade and industrial education, which includes the needle trades, carpentry, drafting, firemen, and similar traditional fields. Other categories are "distributive occupations," meaning selling and retailing, practical nursing, and fishing. . . .

The limitation of Federal aid to rigid occupational categories is a great mistake. One result is that no Federal funds are available for instruction in typing, filing, stenography, and other office work, a field employing ten million people. Similarly the many service jobs which are ideal fields for less gifted students are too avant-garde to receive Federal vo-ed support.

But even if freed from these straitjackets, vo-ed as now consti-tuted cannot prepare students for real jobs. So archaic is most of the training given in vocational schools that unions in the printing, plumbing, food, and other trades refuse to give credit for it. Gradu-ates of vocational schools must start from scratch on apprenticeships often running from three to five years.

Small wonder that a penetrating survey by the Taconic Founda-tion . . . concluded that "it is extremely questionable and certainly has never been demonstrated whether the training absorbed by vo-cational high school graduates is useful to them in getting employ-ment and advancing on the job."

In part this dismal record reflects the extreme difficulty of re-cruiting competent vo-ed teachers (apart from the vo-ags [farming specialists] and homemade pie bakers). City vocational high schools have come to be increasingly thought of as dumping grounds for morons and delinquents—between a third and two thirds of whom vanish before graduating. Most vo-ed teachers are at the bottom of the pedagogic hierarchy. Often they are not even allowed to join the regular teachers' associations. Lacking prestige in a society that esteems the white-collar professions, the blue-collar teachers became identified over the years with the dropouts and washouts—the school failures.

Some years ago, the vo-ed lobby began to worry about this stigma, which, they foresaw, might jeopardize their future slice of the school tax pie. The solution they chose was not the difficult but socially vital one—of reshaping their programs to meet the needs of the majority of students. Instead they began to upgrade their clientele by tightening admissions standards. The less promising were shunted off into the "general curriculum" of academic high schools to pass the time and learn virtually nothing.

Curiously, there has been almost no public outcry against this antisocial policy. Instead, for example, . . . [a 1962] report of the State Education Department on the New York City schools smugly and typically observes that "admissions to programs of skilled trade education should be limited to those students who, on the basis of interest, aptitude, and ability give promise of succeeding."

What then is to happen to the less promising—to the one million jobless out-of-school youth whose ranks . . . [are expected to swell in the years ahead]? Even if some kind of Youth Conservation Corps succeeds in Congress, it will at first serve only 15,000 boys. And what is to become of the millions of adults who, because of the pace of technology and automation, must expect to work at a half dozen different kinds of jobs in a lifetime? These questions are unanswerable in vo-ed's anachronistic terms. But some new answers will have to be found if the new manpower retraining program is to come close to its objective—which is, in essence, the rehabilitation of our hard-core unemployed. As never before in its sheltered history, vo-ed is in the limelight. . . .

## A Workable Formula

The chief handicap of unemployable young people and adults today is not necessarily lack of intelligence. Often it is lack of functional literacy (ability to read at the fifth-grade level). In Chicago a substantial number of relief clients have been able to find work after receiving basic instruction in reading and writing at evening and summer classes sponsored by the city welfare department. Elsewhere it has been found that young people brought up in city slums who drop out of schools geared to middle-class children are not necessarily stupid. And often they are extremely responsive to realistic job training, linked with actual work experience.

This can be accomplished in several ways. About 5 per cent of our colleges now offer what are known as cooperative or work-study education programs. Similar programs exist in academic high schools, chiefly in the business education departments for girls.

Often one job is shared by two trainees, one of whom works for part of the year while the other is at school; on graduating, almost all the trainees get jobs with the companies involved. But except for sales training and in new locally devised schemes, such programs are the exception in vo-ed. Instead, the Federal reimbursement formula requires that students' time be divided concurrently and equally between "practical" (shop) and "related" (academic) classwork—a ritual often unworkable for the many students who can't be taught in classrooms. Frustrated, they drop out. (Labor Secretary [W. Willard] Wirtz aptly calls them "pushouts.")

What is most urgent is that business and labor unions alter their stance in the new age of technological unemployment. The business system is, after all, on trial more than any other institution. It must bear part of the novel social costs arising from technological change with a new resourcefulness and awareness of changing social needs. As a basic starting point, management and the unions must expand apprenticeship programs. Instead of expanding, they have grown steadily smaller (231,000 apprentices in 1950, 166,000 in 1960). Labor must also end its racial discrimination in apprenticeships and abandon its old myopic view that by obstructing entry into the trade—entry being the very thing most necessary for our floating unemployed youth—it will be possible to guarantee jobs for insiders. One of the important breakthroughs of the past year was by New York Local 3 of the International Brotherhood of Electrical Workers. It enrolled two hundred Negroes and Puerto Ricans in its thousand-man training program. Far more unions should be moving in this direction.

Furthermore, business must develop programs for retraining both its own employees and youth in or just out of school. This was the chief lesson which emerged from a National Committee on Employment of Youth conference which I attended recently. Several businessmen observed smugly that a high school diploma is becoming meaningless because their companies' employment standards are so high. "These young graduates can't even qualify for our company training," said a banker. A school superintendent, Mary E. Meade, leaped to her feet. A large, wonderfully plain, almost

Victorian figure of the no-nonsense breed, she is in charge of New York City's minute but highly successful work-study project. This program, financed by the Ford Foundation, enables some high school students to get work experience in municipal government jobs. Miss Meade suggested that maybe business should alter its attitude toward the young and join with the schools in preparing them for useful work. This is still a novel idea although, to be sure, in a few places—all too few—business is beginning to assume some responsibility for training and retraining at least its own workers. The most exciting venture is the new plan developed by the Kaiser Steel Corporation and the United Steelworkers of America. Each worker displaced by automation is placed in a pool, where his wages continue, and he is then either given a new job or is retrained for one within the company. He is not abandoned; he is the company's responsibility until he retires—unless the company suffers grave loss of business or actually folds.

Those who are fainthearted about the possibilities of solving our worsening manpower problems through vocational education and retraining should acquaint themselves with what has been accomplished in rehabilitating the physically disabled—the maimed and paralyzed. In 1961 more than 100,000 disabled people entered gainful employment as a result of the state-Federal program which cost $17 million. Before retraining they had been earning $47 million a year; now they are earning $205 million, and the Federal Government will collect ten dollars in income taxes for each dollar invested in rehabilitation.

This is wonderful. But the best therapy is always preventive. So far as manpower is concerned, the place to start is with the transformation of our system of vocational education. . . .

### Allentown to Denver

In a few isolated spots, there is convincing evidence that vocational training really can work. In Allentown, for instance, local industries cooperate closely with the schools in an outstanding vocational program. Milwaukee, which puts more money into vo-ed than any other city its size, has a model central vocational school.

Cincinnati has dealt with the dropout problem by establishing fourteen vocational training centers throughout the city. Denver's Griffith Opportunity School is a celebrated "skill center" offering free instruction to students of any age.

In these cities, vocational education has, for various reasons, become a matter of major local concern and is vigorously supported by the community. Such sporadic local achievements are widely and justly publicized But this acclaim is unfortunate if it diverts attention from the central fact, namely this: Unless interest in vocational education is awakened on a massive national scale, the United States will lose a crucial lap in "the race between education and catastrophe"—in H. G. Wells's annually more apt definition of history.

Unemployment is both a prime cause and a symptom of the country's alarming economic torpor. Recent economic studies, stemming from the work of Arthur Burns of the National Bureau of Economic Research and from the University of Chicago's Milton Friedman, demonstrate that investment in education rivals investment in physical capital (factories, machinery) in stimulating economic growth. Walter Heller, chairman of the Council of Economic Advisers, has said that such investment in "human capital" has accounted for half of our economic growth in the twentieth century.

Now this hardly seems too difficult a concept for the American people or even Congress to grasp and to act upon. But maybe homelier considerations can be more compelling: the fact, for example, that the loss in production in the United States caused by unemployment in 1962 was greater than the loss caused by the strikes in the last thirty-five years; or that, to the average man, the loss of only one year's income due to unemployment is more than the total cost of twelve years of education through high school. However one may dramatize the issue, the essential point is that education, employment, and economic growth are inextricably linked. Today rational education must include training pertinent for the 80 per cent of all young Americans who enter the labor market without college degrees. To ignore their vocational training is a reverse twist on the Eskimos' fabled custom of pushing their unproductive senior citizens onto the ice pack. That practice at least has a certain economic logic. Our system is managing to be at once inhumane and economically suicidal.

## THE IMBALANCE IN EDUCATIONAL OPPORTUNITY [3]

The Civil Rights Act of 1964 contains a section numbered 402, which went largely unnoticed at the time. This section instructs the Commissioner of Education to carry out a survey "concerning the lack of availability of equal educational opportunities" by reason of race, religion or national origin, and to report to Congress and the President within two years. The congressional intent in this section is somewhat unclear. But if, as is probable, the survey was initially intended as a means of finding areas of continued intentional discrimination, the intent later became less punitive-oriented and more future-oriented: i.e., to provide a basis for public policy, at the local, state, and national levels, which might overcome inequalities of educational opportunity.

In the two years that have intervened (but mostly in the second), a remarkably vast and comprehensive survey was conducted, focusing principally on the inequalities of educational opportunity experienced by five racial and ethnic minorities: Negroes, Puerto Ricans, Mexican Americans, American Indians, and Oriental Americans. In the central and largest portion of the survey, nearly 600,000 children at grades 1, 3, 6, 9, and 12, in 4,000 schools in all fifty states and the District of Columbia, were tested and questioned; 60,000 teachers in these schools were questioned and self-tested; and principals of these schools were also questioned about their schools. The tests and questionnaires (administered in the fall of 1965 by Educational Testing Service) raised a considerable controversy in public school circles and among some parents, with concern ranging from Federal encroachment on the local education system to the specter of invasion of privacy. Nevertheless, with a participation rate of about 70 per cent of all the schools sampled, the survey was conducted; and on July 1, 1966, Commissioner Howe presented a

[3] From "Equal Schools or Equal Students?" by James S. Coleman, professor of social relations at Johns Hopkins University. *Public Interest.* no 4:70-5. Summer '66. Reprinted by permission.

summary report of this survey. On July 31, the total report, *Equality of Educational Opportunity,* 737 pages, was made available. . . .

Perhaps the greatest virtue of this survey—though it has many faults—is that it did not take a simple or politically expedient view of educational opportunity. To have done so would have meant to measure (a) the objective characteristics of schools—number of books in the library, age of buildings, educational level of teachers, accreditation of the schools, and so on; and (b) the actual extent of racial segregation in the schools. The survey did look into these matters (and found less inequity in school facilities and resources, more in the extent of segregation, than is commonly supposed); but its principal focus of attention was not on what resources go into education, but on what product comes out. It did this in a relatively uncomplicated way, which is probably adequate for the task at hand: by tests which measured those areas of achievement most necessary for further progress in school, in higher education, and in successful competition in the labor market—that is, verbal and reading skills, and analytical and mathematical skills. Such a criterion does not allow statements about absolute levels of inequality or equality of education provided by the schools, because obviously there are more influences than the school's on a child's level of achievement in school, and there are more effects of schools than in these areas of achievement. What it does do is to broaden the question beyond the school to all those educational influences that have their results in the level of verbal and mathematical skill a young person is equipped wth when he or she enters the adult world. In effect, it takes the perspective of this young adult, and says that what matters to him is, not how "equal" his school is, but rather whether he is equipped at the end of school to compete on an equal basis with others, whatever his social origins. From the perspective of society, it assumes that what is important is not to equalize the schools in some formal sense, but to insure that children from all groups come into adult society so equipped as to insure their full participation in this society.

Another way of putting this is to say that the schools are successful only insofar as they reduce the dependence of a child's opportunities upon his social origins. We can think of a set of conditional probabilities: the probability of being prepared for a given occupation or for a given college at the end of high school, conditional upon the child's social origins. The effectiveness of the schools consists, in part, of making the conditional probabilities less conditional—that is, less dependent upon social origins. Thus, equality of educational opportunity implies, not merely "equal" schools, but equally effective schools, whose influences will overcome the differences in starting point of children from different social groups.

## The Widening Educational Gap

This approach to educational opportunity, using as it does achievement on standardized tests, treads on sensitive ground. Differences in average achievement between racial groups can lend themselves to racist arguments of genetic differences in intelligence; even apart from this, they can lead to invidious comparisons between groups which show different average levels of achievement. But it is precisely the avoidance of such sensitive areas that can perpetuate the educational deficiencies with which some minorities are equipped at the end of schooling.

What, then, does the survey find with regard to effects of schooling on test achievement? Children were tested at the beginning of grades 1, 3, 6, 9, and 12. Achievement of the average American Indian, Mexican American, Puerto Rican, and Negro (in this descending order) was much lower than the average white or Oriental American, at all grade levels. The amount of difference ranges from about half a standard deviation to one standard deviation at early grade levels. At the twelfth grade, it increases to beyond one standard deviation. (One standard deviation difference means that about 85 per cent of the minority group children score below the average of the whites, while if the groups were equal only about 50 per cent would score below this average.) The grade levels of difference range up to five years of deficiency (in math achievement) or four years (in reading skills) at the twelfth grade. In short, the differences are large to begin with, and they are even larger at higher grades.

Two points, then, are clear: (1) these minority children have a serious educational deficiency at the start of school, which is obviously not a result of school; and (2) they have an even more serious deficiency at the end of school, which is obviously in part a result of school.

Thus, by the criterion stated earlier—that the effectiveness of schools in creating equality of educational opportunity lies in making the conditional probabilities of success less conditional—the schools appear to fail. At the end of school, the conditional probabilities of high achievement are even more conditional upon racial or ethnic background than they are at the beginning of school.

There are a number of results from the survey which give further evidence on this matter. First, within each racial group, the strong relation of family economic and educational background to achievement does not diminish over the period of school, and may even increase over the elementary years. Second, most of the variation in student achievement lies within the same school, very little of it is between schools. The implication of these last two results is clear: family background differences account for much more variation in achievement than do school differences.

Even the school-to-school variation in achievement, though relatively small, is itself almost wholly due to the *social* environment provided by the school: the educational backgrounds and aspirations of other students in the school, and the educational backgrounds and attainments of the teachers in the school. Per pupil expenditure, books in the library, and a host of other facilities and curricular measures show virtually no relation to achievement if the "social" environment of the school—the educational backgrounds of other students and teachers—is held constant.

The importance of this last result lies, of course, in the fact that schools, as currently organized, are quite culturally homogeneous as well as quite racially segregated: teachers tend to come from the same cultural groups (and especially from the same race) as their students, and the student bodies are themselves relatively homogeneous. Given this homogeneity, the principal agents of effectiveness in the schools—teachers and other students—act to maintain or reinforce the initial differences imposed by social origins.

One element illustrates well the way in which the current organization of schools maintains the differences over generations: a Negro prospective teacher leaves a Negro teachers' college with a much lower level of academic competence (as measured by the National Teacher's Examination) than does his white counterpart leaving his largely white college; then he teaches Negro children (in school with other Negro children, ordinarily from educationally deficient backgrounds), who learn at a lower level, in part because of his lesser competence; some of these students, in turn, go into teacher training institutions to become poorly-trained teachers of the next generation.

Altogether, the sources of inequality of educational opportunity appear to lie first in the home itself and the cultural influences immediately surrounding the home; then they lie in the schools' ineffectiveness to free achievement from the impact of the home, and in the schools' cultural homogeneity which perpetuates the social influences of the home and its environs.

### A Modest, Yet Radical Proposal

Given these results, what do they suggest as to avenues to equality of educational opportunity? Several elements seem clear:

(a) For those children whose family and neighborhood are educationally disadvantaged, it is important to replace this family environment as much as possible with an educational environment —by starting school at an earlier age, and by having a school which begins very early in the day and ends very late.

(b) It is important to reduce the social and racial homogeneity of the school environment, so that those agents of education that do show some effectiveness—teachers and other students—are not mere replicas of the student himself. In the present organization of schools, it is the neighborhood school that most insures such homogeneity.

(c) The educational program of the school should be made more effective than it is at present. The weakness of this program is apparent in its inability to overcome initial differences. It is hard to believe that we are so inept in educating our young that we can do no more than leave young adults in the same relative competitive positions we found them in as children.

Several points are obvious: It is not a solution simply to pour money into improvement of the physical plants, books, teaching aids, of schools attended by educationally disadvantaged children. For other reasons, it will not suffice merely to bus children or otherwise achieve pro forma integration. (One incidental effect of this would be to increase the segregation within schools, through an increase in tracking.) [Tracking, in educational jargon, means separating children for instruction according to ability.—Ed.]

The only kinds of policies that appear in any way viable are those which do not seek to improve the education of Negroes and other educationally disadvantaged at the expense of those who are educationally advantaged. This implies new kinds of educational institutions, with a vast increase in expenditures for education—not merely for the disadvantaged, but for all children. The solutions might be in the form of educational parks, or in the form of private schools paid by tuition grants (with Federal regulations to insure racial heterogeneity), public (or publicly subsidized) boarding schools (like the North Carolina Advancement School), or still other innovations. This approach also implies reorganization of the curriculum within schools. One of the major reasons for tracking is the narrowness of our teaching methods—they can tolerate only a narrow range of skill in the same classroom. Methods which greatly widen the range are necessary to make possible racial and cultural integration within a school—and thus to make possible the informal learning that other students of higher educational levels can provide. Such curricular innovations are possible—but, again, only through the investment of vastly greater sums in education than currently occurs.

It should be recognized, of course, that the goal described here—of equality of educational opportunity through the schools—is far more ambitious than has ever been posed in our society before. The schools were once seen as a supplement to the family in bringing a child into his place in adult society, and they still function largely as such a supplement, merely perpetuating the inequalities of birth. Yet the conditions imposed by technological change, and by our postindustrial society, quite apart from any ideals of equal opportunity, require a far more primary role for the school, if society's children are to be equipped for adulthood.

## Self-Confidence and Performance

One final result of the survey gives an indication of still another —and perhaps the most important—element necessary for equality of educational opportunity for Negroes. One attitude of students was measured at grades 9 and 12—an attitude which indicated the degree to which the student felt in control of his own fate. For example, one question was: "Agree or disagree: good luck is more important than hard work for success." Another was: "Agree or disagree: every time I try to get ahead someone or something stops me." Negroes much less often than whites had such a sense of control of their fate—a difference which corresponds directly to reality, and which corresponds even more markedly to the Negro's historical position in American society. However, despite the very large achievement differences between whites and Negroes at the ninth and twelfth grades, those Negroes who gave responses indicating a sense of control of their own fate achieved higher on the tests than those whites who gave the opposite responses. This attitude was more highly related to achievement than any other factor in the students' background or school.

This result suggests that internal changes in the Negro, changes in his conception of himself in relation to his environment, may have more effect on Negro achievement than any other single factor. The determination to overcome relevant obstacles, and the belief that he will overcome them—attitudes that have appeared in an organized way among Negroes only in recent years in some civil rights groups—may be the most crucial elements in achieving equality of opportunity—not because of changes they will create in the white community, but principally because of the changes they create in the Negro himself.

## SCHOOLS AS SOCIAL INSTRUMENTS: A CRITIQUE [4]

All across the nation this fact is beginning to stand out:

It is the average young American who is becoming the neglected and almost forgotten generation of today.

Vast and growing sums of public and private funds are showering down on the dull youngster, the dropout, the delinquent—and those whom the sociologists call the culturally deprived young people of America.

At the other extreme, children of the well-to-do, or youngsters with very high intelligence quotients, are getting access to well-staffed private schools, scholarships and other aids on their way to top colleges and choice careers.

Left in the middle, without benefit of private privilege or of tax-supported bounties, is the great bulk of young persons of ordinary means and talent.

These are the average children, coming mostly from middle-class families, who usually stay out of serious trouble, manage to "get by" in their studies, and seem to have few anxieties. Many are going on to college—but even more are planning to settle down to jobs and marriage unless drafted.

Such youngsters, in the past, were considered the backbone of America's future. Through successive generations, the average youngsters have contributed much of America's leadership—in recent times such men as Harry Truman, Dwight D. Eisenhower and Lyndon B. Johnson.

Now it is no longer the average child who is the focus of the nation's concern for its youth. Instead, money and attention are being turned to the child at either extreme.

### Wooing the Disadvantaged

Special care is being lavished on the disadvantaged child—all the way from cradle to adulthood.

[4] From "The Forgotten Youth in Today's America." *U.S. News & World Report.* 60:52-4+. F. 21, '66. Reprinted from *U.S. News & World Report*, published at Washington.

Many of these youngsters are born onto welfare rolls. Today they are going to preschool nurseries designed especially to make them feel less disadvantaged when they enter school.

If a youngster somehow fails to respond to this help, youth agencies are on hand to provide him with advice, recreation or psychotherapy.

Should that fail, the dropout or delinquent is sought out by the Job Corps with offers of free room, board and spending money if he will consent to finish his schooling and go to work.

The bright child, too, is getting a full measure of the nation's solicitude at this time.

Such youngsters are being watched over and pushed ahead, grade by grade. For these children there are competitions for science awards, for scholarships to "name" colleges, and even appearances on television quiz contests. Corporation executives scan college grades and bid for services of top grades. Book publishers give wide publicity to "alienated" and "sensitive" boys and girls who have sad stories to tell—and sell—about their sufferings.

In contrast, the lot of the middle-range youngster is seen as rather drab. One teacher said:

"The only agency I know of that has a fond interest in the average kid is the draft board. And that's only because the armed forces don't want the dull student, and can't get at the bright student because of his grades."

Increasingly, complaints are being heard about the quality of education being given the average student. In Detroit's suburbs, one mother said:

"Maybe my son isn't a brain, but he's just as entitled to good teachers as anyone else. He needs to get all he can out of high school because he may not qualify for college."

In the same suburb, a father complained that his son's school was geared heavily to the college-bound student.

"About the only thing left to my son is auto shop—but he isn't a mechanic and never could be," this father said.

In Houston, Bob Eckels, chairman of the school board, is urging "more emphasis on the 80 per cent who are either going to carry us forward or let us go broke in the future."

Average youngsters are taking note of their situation.

In Seattle, a University of Washington senior is seeking to raise $150,000 to help "just average" high school graduates attend college. The student, Anthony Valdez, said he launched his campaign because he was forced to enter the Army several years ago for lack of funds to go to college. He said:

"Why shouldn't deserving students who graduate from high school with average grades and insufficient funds be given a scholarship? Their value to the community can be increased if they are given a chance to go to college or vocational school."

## "Brains," "Kooks" and Counselors

On a high school level, a seventeen-year-old boy in Prince Georges County, a suburb of Washington, D.C., said:

"Our counselors have mass meetings with the students and parents at the beginning of the school.

"They always say, 'Feel free to come to me at any time with your individual problem.' But they manage to give me the impression that they're far too busy to be bothered with me unless I've got some kind of a real hang-up. So the great majority of kids like me, who aren't doing too badly anyway, just never visit the counselor and our parents don't either."

This boy, who is on the track and field team and has a better-than-C average, said he might go on to college. But he added:

"It's not easy, you know. If some 'brain' gets a science award, or some 'kook' paints a dirty word on the wall, they'll have their way all taken care of. But I can't find time in the school day to get into the office when the counselor's around. If I did, I'd be in trouble for skipping class."

What is taking place, as many educators see it, is a basic shift in the schools—away from the idea of school as a collection of youngsters, and toward the concept that the school is really a "social instrument" and that children are to be treated according to whatever "social group" they fit into.

Dr. Mark Bills, superintendent of public schools in Peoria, Ill., said:

> The major problem and threat to American education right now is an almost frenzied emphasis on "equalization," on cultural background, on sociological climate.
>
> If you have to point an educational program toward those with lower abilities, the other students just have to go along on their own. This makes it difficult for the middle group especially. Only the cream of the students can get along well without close attention and guidance from teachers.

### How Federal Aid Figures

The vast program of Federal aid to education, approved last year by Congress, is seen by many educators as accelerating the trend toward use of the school as a "social instrument."

About three quarters of all funds authorized for helping public schools was earmarked for low-income districts, which have the highest percentages of dull students.

Low-income students of average or less ability got $58 million for college "scholarships" with no repayment required. For the middle-income student, a guaranteed-loan program was provided. This makes it easier for the student to get a loan, and he is relieved of interest payments until he finishes school. But in most cases the loan must be repaid by him or his parents—who often are hard pressed to get several youngsters through college on moderate incomes.

The backward child, especially if he lives in the slums, is getting other help from the Government.

During the . . . [1965-66] school year, the "war on poverty" is making $188 million available for preschool training for "disadvantaged" youngsters. Another 700 millions is earmarked for programs containing provisions for education of the poor, such as the Job Corps.

On the other end of the scale, incentives are being provided for "gifted" youngsters through federally aided research on accelerated studies and "enrichment" programs.

Backed by these types of Federal aid, local school systems are launching a wide variety of programs aimed at the "exceptional" child. In many instances, school boards are under pressure from racial minorities to give favored treatment to "disadvantaged" children.

In New York, for instance, millions are being spent—with the help of Federal funds and foundation grants—on training teachers for slum areas, setting up preschool nurseries for the poor, busing Negro youngsters to predominantly white schools and providing special textbooks for the slow learners.

In addition, New York is spending heavily on the education of the bright child. Quick learners are channeled into special classes at the elementary level, and can go on to one of several high schools for the brilliant.

Similarly, across the continent, classrooms in San Francisco's low-income districts tend to have three or four fewer pupils per teacher than is the case of middle-income areas—while bright students also get special attention with the help of state grants for the education of "gifted" children.

As another example, Pittsburgh has set up a "division of compensatory education" aimed especially at uplifting Negro youngsters. "Undermotivated" children from low-income neighborhoods are being sought out and encouraged to go on to college—and there is also a "scholar's program" to push along the brightest students in the city.

## A Dubious Trickle?

It is the contention of many educators that such programs are not hurting, and may even be helping the average student. Benefits tailored to the bright and the dull, it is held, trickle down to the middle-range child.

Doubts, however, are beginning to arise about this viewpoint. Even the track system, which is supposed to separate children according to ability, is coming under fire. In Washington, D.C., a white parent complained:

"Teachers feel that it's exciting to work with honors kids, and a challenge to try to teach something to the backward child—or, if they don't feel the challenge, the minorities are ready to jump down their throats. The trouble is, nobody feels the prestige or challenge of working with an average kid, so it is pretty easy to tuck him away in the college-prep or general track on a 'file and forget' basis."

In a Chicago suburb, a teacher in an elementary school said:

"I notice that most of the afterschool programs and extracurricular activities seem to be for either the bright or the dull students. In the classroom, you have to give more attention to the slower learners. Sometimes, when I'm making out grades, I come to a name and say to myself: 'Mary—Mary who?' I've forgotten all about her. She's an average student."

A Houston educator, rejecting the claim that average students are benefiting from the emphasis on exceptional youngsters, said: "If you have all the extras for the particularly high student, or the particularly low student, you're taking it out of the hides of the teachers and students in the average group."

Also developing is worry that growing emphasis on the culturally deprived children is leading to an acceptance of questionable values in the schools. One Brooklyn educator, for example, is calling on teachers to recognize such "lower-class values as energy, spontaneity and direct-sense gratification." The latter term was not defined, but some critics asked if using switch-blade knives is a "direct-sense gratification." . . .

Fear of some psychologists is that "lower-class values," once given a place in school systems, will "reach out" for average children, too. An official of the National Institutes of Health, Thomas Gladwin, has warned school officials against what he described as growing cynicism about "middle-class values"—gentility, hard work and planning for the future.

At this time, the prevailing trend is toward even more help for the exceptional child, especially if he is backward and comes from a background of poverty.

Francis Keppel, . . . named Assistant Secretary of Health, Education, and Welfare [in September 1965], made this comment as United States Commissioner of Education when asked about what could be done for the problem students from comfortable homes:

I say bluntly that these are not the first concern in my mind as the United States Commissioner of Education. These kids eat well. Or, if they don't eat well, it's their own fault. If they don't have a decent and human kind of relationship with their parents, it is to a degree their fault. . . . I am much more concerned with those of whom it can clearly be said that deprivation is not their fault, or even that of their parents.

Of course I have great sympathy for these students from affluent homes. These adolescents are under great pressure for success, measured in middle-class values—the values which the upper class looks down on and the lower class looks down on, too. These children have a sense of pressure—are they going to get into college as their mothers and fathers did? This pressure now is greater on them than it was in their fathers' and mothers' generation. Some of these youngsters are breaking and bending under the pressure and we ought to show Christian compassion and human sympathy for them. But while they are having a tough time they aren't anywhere as badly off as the others, the deprived 20 per cent.

## An $8.4 Billion View

This viewpoint comes from the top Federal official dealing directly with the schools—and the impact of his views on the entire future of American schools can be measured by the fact that Federal spending on education in the next fiscal year is likely to reach nearly $8.4 billion, or close to one fifth of all the nation's spending on education. [In April 1966 Mr. Keppel left the Department of Health, Education, and Welfare to become president and chairman of the board of directors of General Learning Corporation.—Ed.]

Some of the nation's top educators are expressing concern over the growing emphasis being placed by schools on the exceptional child and what this may be doing to the quality of education offered the middle-range youngster.

Dr. Harold Spears, San Francisco's school superintendent, plans a major campaign on behalf of average students when he assumes presidency of the American Association of School Administrators. . . .

This authority is pointing out that preschool training for the poor is, in effect, a "means test" which excludes middle-class children. His prediction:

"Middle-class parents will be hammering at school boards all over the nation to get the same kind of help for their children— and I believe they ought to get it."

At a recent meeting of California school administrators he said:

This is not the day of the average in school. It is the period of the different—the exceptional—of distinctions. Both the state legislature and Congress, in dispensing school funds, are packaging the stuff in the manner of the druggist handling prescriptions, each shipment indicating a specific patient and the dosage.

Perhaps there's nothing more humiliating than to be an average student, with an IQ of 100, who gets his lessons, causes no disturbance, has a girl friend, isn't in an honors course, has never been in the principal's office, isn't asking for his rights, goes out for football instead of a merit scholarship, doesn't have a counselor tailing him from morning 'til night—and doesn't realize he needs one.

If we can judge by the trend in legislative action, pretty soon the average student will run the danger of being "discovered" and then classified as a misfit, not belonging to the "in" group—that is, the group in the legislature's mind at the moment.

When this happens he will lose his privacy. But you can be sure that he will in turn inherit a rich legacy of public funds.

## III. IMPACT OF THE FEDERAL GOVERNMENT

## EDITOR'S INTRODUCTION

Civil rights enforcement, the war on poverty and Great Society concern with education in general have over the past half decade thrust the Federal Government into the vanguard of educational reform. Today the Department of Health, Education, and Welfare under Secretary John W. Gardner and the United States Office of Education under Harold Howe II are involved in a host of programs and projects designed to upgrade, equalize, and expand. The children of the poor have thus far been the primary beneficiaries of Federal assistance, but Washington's role may be expected to have a wide-ranging impact.

Just as war is too important a matter to be left to the generals, so—Washington seems to have concluded—education is too important a matter to be left to the educators. One facet of the new Federal involvement is to bring new kinds of people into activity at the local school level—musicians, artists, writers, businessmen and others with practical experience in various fields of endeavor. Supplementary Educational Centers are being established to make television programs, teach subjects not taught in the local curriculum, establish specialized vocational training programs and in general make "nuisances" of themselves in terms of goading local community action. Though the old argument that Federal aid means Federal control seems to have been put to rest by the passage of the Elementary and Secondary Education Act of 1965, there is no reason to suppose that clashes between local and Federal authorities will not grow apace with increasing Federal involvement. There is, in fact, a growing body of complaints against Federal "interference," as the last article in this section makes clear.

This section seeks to draw a broad outline of the Federal Government's impact on our nation's schools. In the first article a writer in the *New Republic* details the revolutionary character of President Johnson's school program and suggests, approvingly, the benefits that may accrue to our school systems as a result. A detailed account of the provisions of the Elementary and Secondary Education Act of 1965, as finally passed by Congress, follows.

The last two articles debate a growing controversy over Federal guidelines in the desegregation process. In the first of these a director of educational research and development at Rhode Island College complains angrily about the slow pace of desegregation and suggests ways in which the process might be speeded up. Criticism of the guidelines and their impact on local school districts from the opposite viewpoint is summarized in the second.

## WASHINGTON SPONSORS A REVOLUTION [1]

It is too early to be sure, but conversation on Capitol Hill suggests that the Administration's education bills are likely to be enacted with only minor amendments. [For an analysis of what finally emerged, see the next article in this section.—Ed.] If so, the result could be a revolution in American education. The proposals for elementary and secondary education are the most far-reaching and radical ever to come from the White House. Instead of simply asking Congress to give the educational establishment more money to continue doing the same things it has done for years, the proposed legislation would attempt to change the ways of that establishment by broadening its political, social and intellectual base. The old feudal pattern of local sovereignty and state regulation, which worked to the disadvantage of the Catholics, the poor and the intellectuals, is at long last to be assaulted. And the assault, instead of being led by political outsiders, will have the fiscal and administrative backing of the Federal Government.

Like all Johnson proposals, the Elementary and Secondary Education Act of 1965 is being promoted with a highly traditional rhetoric. The authors have even written a provision forbidding Fed-

[1] From "LBJ's School Program: A Revolution in American Education?" by Christopher Jencks, contributing editor. *New Republic.* 152:17-20. F. 6, '65. Reprinted by permission of *The New Republic,* copyright 1965, Harrison-Blaine of New Jersey, Inc.

eral "direction, supervision or control" over any aspect of education. Nevertheless, anyone who looks carefully at the bill will see that it represents a major indictment of the educational system as managed by state and local boards of education and school superintendents, and that it proposes to remedy many of their failures by substituting the political judgments and academic priorities of the Congress and the United States Commissioner of Education.

So far as the President is concerned, the most important failure of the state and local authorities seems to be the combination of incompetence and indifference which has excluded the poor from many of the benefits of public education. This failure is beginning to have serious political consequences. The Democratic party has since 1929 had the overwhelming support of the blue-collar classes. The party's ability to retain this support, and to contain the nascent extremism and violence in this group, has depended in good part on providing schooling which led to jobs and a chance for at least a few to move up in the world, Today the schools are not doing that job, and the explosive consequences are increasingly obvious— especially in the Negro ghettoes. Unemployment and violence threaten to undermine the coalition of ethnic minorities which has been one of the primary sources of Democratic voting strength.

The basic reasons for the school's failure to do what needs to be done for the poor are clear. Education has become largely a competitive sport, valued by the public because it can set their children apart from others and ensure them a larger share of wealth and power. There are only a limited number of places in the "top" colleges and professional schools, and only a finite number of jobs which provide generous salaries and a chance to exercise responsibility. Competition for these openings is rough, and even the most enlightened parent will fight to ensure his children a more than "equal" chance at them; *his* children must attend the "best" schools, be they public or private. Such ambitions mean that every time the public schools in a neighboring district are improved, the public schools in one's own district have to be improved equally— or a little more. Hence although middle-class parents seldom consciously oppose improving schools which serve the poor, they do resist efforts to narrow the gap between these schools and those which serve their own children.

## The Children of the Poor

The most obvious example is found in the formulas by which legislatures have allocated state aid money to local school districts. Traditionally, these formulas were rigged to give special help to poor rural districts, which had large numbers of representatives in state legislatures. Urban areas got back less state aid than they contributed in state taxes. In recent years however, many state aid formulas have been revised, usually at the behest of professional educators, to reward districts which live up to or exceed certain "minimal" standards of performance set by the state department of education. This "incentive" system has often benefited wealthy districts, especially suburban ones, while penalizing poor districts which can meet minimal standards only by heroic tax effort. The reapportionment of state legislatures will presumably accelerate this tendency, since for the most part it will give the rich suburbanites more votes and the dwindling farmers fewer.

Against this background the Administration's proposals look courageous. Out of $1.25 billion to be spent on elementary and secondary education in fiscal 1965-66, the President is asking that $1 billion go directly to help the children of the poor. The formula for allocating Federal funds would be based on the number of children in each school district whose families had annual incomes of less than $2,000. For each such child a district would receive a payment equal to half the average per-pupil expenditure in the state. This formula would enable Mississippi, for example, to increase its current school expenditures by about 20 per cent, while a state like California could spend only about 3 per cent more. It would also mean that when Mississippi got its check from Washington it would have to allocate the money to local districts on a basis which corresponds at least crudely with need, rather than with political influence.

The difference between this proposal and the "general aid" programs vainly submitted to Congress by Presidents Kennedy,

Eisenhower and Truman is a measure both of the political impact of last November's elections and of Lyndon Johnson's genius in making antipoverty programs seem respectable. Earlier proposals for general aid to education were primarily intended to shift part of the cost of local schools from the state sales taxes and local property taxes to Federal income taxes. This meant a shift from mildly regressive to mildly progressive taxes, but that was by no means the major purpose of the proposals; their aim was to increase the total burden of education taxes on everyone. In addition, the proposal sought to include some kind of "equalization" formula which would give the poor southern and mountain states more money per pupil than the rich states of the East and West coasts. But again, "equalization" was never the fundamental objective; it was a gimmick whose main purpose was to make a controversial proposal attractive to wavering southerners. The basic indifference of the proponents of general aid to equalization was indicated by their unanimous readiness to let state legislators allocate Federal funds among local school districts according to any formula they liked, be it progressive or regressive.

## The Contest: Rich Versus Poor

If I am right in suggesting that education is in large part a competitive enterprise, what may be shaping up is a contest in which the middle classes try to use their control over state and local government to get more money for their own schools, while the poor use whatever political and emotional leverage they have on the Federal Government to get more for theirs. Whether the result of this contest will be to widen or narrow the gap between rich and poor will depend on whether the White House plays for keeps or only for show. The constitutional and fiscal powers of the Federal Government are more than sufficient to prevent state and local powers being used for the selfish ends of a single class, but the rhetoric of "local control" may prevent these powers from being used.

The battle, if there is to be one, will probably be joined over state aid formulas. The Johnson education bill would forbid any state to revise its formula so as to offset the effect of the proposed Federal legislation. This provision was inserted to prevent state legislatures from doing what many have done with regard to Federal assistance for "impacted areas," namely reducing the state aid to which a district is entitled by the amount it gets from Washington. The long-term problem is not, however, to prevent states from reducing their aid to poor areas. It is to prevent their raising payments to rich districts faster than Washington raises payments to poor ones. If a state revises its aid formula to reward districts which are already doing a good job, instead of trying to help those which are doing badly because of an inadequate tax base, will Federal assistance to the state be cut? Not if the President is Lyndon Johnson—though the wording of the proposed legislation might seem to require it.

## *Upgrading Parochial Schools*

President Johnson's efforts to make the public schools serve the poor as well as the prosperous have been matched by a somewhat less wholehearted effort to make them serve Catholics as well as non-Catholics. Half the Catholic children in America now attend parochial schools, and on paper these schools bear a marked resemblance to the slum schools on which so much concern is now being focused. Parochial schools are usually housed in older buildings than public schools, their classes larger, their textbooks more outmoded, their teachers worse paid and worse prepared, their libraries less adequate. Yet it may be doubted whether President Johnson's concern with Catholic education derived from such statistics. Nor is there any reason why it should have done so. While parochial schools may have some of the external attributes of slum schools, a recent survey by Andrew Greeley, Peter Rossi and Leonard Pinto of the University of Chicago shows that they mostly cater to very different sorts of children. Catholics who attend parochial schools come from wealthier and better educated families than Catholics who attend public schools. Ethnically, parochial school families are likely to trace their ancestry back to the "old" rather than the "new" immigrants, to countries in Northern Europe which had been exposed to the mixed blessings of Protestantism rather than to Mediterranean countries which had not. Italian, Puerto Rican and Mexican Catholics seem to have a particularly marked allergy to sending their children to parochial schools, while French and Irish Catholics are the parochial schools' most loyal supporters. Yet even when these differences are taken into account, and parochial school Catholics are compared to socially similar Catholics who attend public school, the survey seems to show that those who attend parochial school are more likely to graduate from secondary school, more likely to attend college, and more likely to land a good job.

Bearing this in mind it is understandable that the Administration should give the improvement of the parochial schools a rather low priority. But the Administration *is* concerned about doing enough for the parochial schools to win support from the Catholic hierarchy for Federal aid to education, or failing that to win at least neutrality. With this in view, the Administration has offered Federal support for whatever portion of Catholic education the hierarchy is willing to place under public control. How much or how little will be left to the prejudices and finances of each parish, and to a lesser extent of each school district. "Dual enrollment," as the new bill rechristens "shared time," may involve nothing more than sending a few parochial school boys to the public school for work in expensive vocational training facilities, or it may mean sending Catholic students to the public school for science, mathematics, foreign languages, vocational training, and even physical exercise. Federal funds will also be available to buy library books and textbooks for parochial schools, but the list of books which can be purchased will be determined by the secular board of education, not by the hierarchy. How far the parochial schools will go in secularizing their texts and libraries remains to be seen. Some have already gone far.

While these proposals are constitutionally and politically sound, they will probably not do as much to narrow the gap between Catholic and non-Catholic as Mr. Johnson hopes to do in narrowing the gap between rich and poor. It is true that Catholics often resent paying ever higher property taxes to support public schools their children do not attend, that such resentment among voters has made improvements in public education increasingly difficult in some communities, and that shared time might be (and sometimes has been) a way around this dilemma. This would be especially true if the principle were extended so that, for example, a remedial reading teacher on the public payroll could spend two mornings a week working in the parochial school, instead of requiring each slow reader in the parochial school to go to the public school for such instruction. But will the proposed Federal program, confined as it is to low-income children, provide enough incentive to force cooperation on public and parochial schools which largely serve middle-class families? In many cases the answer will probably be no. If Washington is going to lead local educators out of their present impasse, it will probably have to go further than it has so far in promoting cooperation. But the Administration's bill is an excellent beginning.

## *Educational Centers*

The third area of Federal innovation, and in many respects the most unsettling to the established system of state and local control, is the effort to bring new kinds of people into local public education. The recent history of this dream goes back to the middle 1950's, when the National Science Foundation and a number of private groups discovered that high school science courses were being taught by men who not only were not scientists but who had not the slightest idea what scientists did. This discovery led to an effort to get working scientists involved in public education, first as curriculum reformers, then as teachers of science teachers, and most recently as part-time teachers of public school students. The prestige of the university scientist was so great that the public schools often felt compelled to accept their advice and assistance, but efforts to generalize the pattern to other subjects were less successful. Washington reformers have been trying to engage musicians in music education, artists in art education, novelists and poets in the teaching of English, and businessmen in vocational training. They have also sought to involve not just the public schools but a wide range of public and quasi-public institutions in the education of the young: colleges and universities, libraries, museums, theaters, newspapers, politicians, and even the League of Women Voters. Such suggestions have seldom been received enthusiastically by local school administrators, who are jealous of their power, skeptical of know-it-all outsiders, and convinced that what they need is more support for what they are already doing, not proposals for new things.

The Administration's efforts to change all this will be conducted through institutions known as Supplementary Educational Centers. These will be financed by grants from the United States Office of Education, and controlled by boards which are supposed to include representatives not only of the local school system but of other relevant institutions. The Centers will be able to do almost anything the Office of Education (or anyone else) gives them money to do: make television programs, set up specialized occupational training programs, provide additional guidance and counseling (whatever that may mean), teach subjects not being taught in the regular public schools, and most important, teach established subjects in new ways. The Centers will be free to hire the uncertified, to use part-time instructors, and to hire people jointly with a university or other institution.

## Cosmopolitan Values?

Whether such institutions can actually germinate a revolution in American education will depend on how they are administered. At worst, the local educators may make only nominal efforts to cooperate with other institutions and individuals in their communities, submitting proposals to Washington which merely call for hiring guidance officers to talk dropouts into sticking it out for another year, or for buying more electronic gadgets nobody knows how to use properly. At best, there will be stiff competition for the $100 million available for these Centers in fiscal 1965-66; the United States Office [of Education] will approve the more daring and radical proposals; and the stodgier school superintendents will get the message and return with more imaginative ideas next year.

Being dependent for survival on their ability to impress Washington with their value to local students, the Centers may feel compelled to try things which the local public schools are reluctant to attempt. They may even become outposts for cosmopolitan values, at least partially immune to the prevailing local orthodoxies and self-satisfactions. If their example is then taken up in the public schools, so much the better. But even if it is not, local students who find the public schools claustrophobic may for the first time have an alternative in the federally sponsored Centers.

Unfortunately, grants for Centers will be evaluated not by the Bureau of the Budget or the Office of Science and Technology, which were largely responsible for getting the Centers into the President's program, but by the United States Office of Education, many of whose officials are as distrustful as local schoolmen of the ideas and individuals behind the Centers. Had the matter been left solely to the Office, the Centers might not even have been included in the Johnson proposals, or at least not in their present promising form.

Indeed, it seems to me that the most serious defect of the whole Johnson program is the fact that it will be administered by people who are partially or completely out of sympathy with its fundamental objectives. Enormous reliance is being placed on the states, and especially on beefed-up state departments of education, which are unprepared for these new tasks. The same is true of many parts of the Office of Education. Leaving almost everything to the states is meant to reassure skeptical Congressmen who are worried (not without reason) about a Federal takeover. But politics are not the only motive. There is no group of men and women anywhere in America ready to run the kind of program which the President's proposals envision. The only alternative to placing power in the hands of the states would be to place it in nobody's hands, at least for the moment. Nevertheless, instead of trying to work through the state departments of education, the Administration might have taken the position (privately) that most state departments are incompetent. A new division of the Office of Education could then have been established, with new men running it. For a year or two this would have meant near anarchy, and much money would have been wasted on projects which the Office had neither the time nor the skill to evaluate. In the long run, a new agency would have been able to draft the talented individuals who will inevitably surface once new programs go into action. The Administration's chosen approach, on the other hand, will place enormous power in the hands of established mediocrities, and will work against the appearance of new men and new ideas. Nor will it prevent waste, for the state education departments are riddled with incompetents who will endorse every bad check presented to them.

Still, for all their limitations, President Johnson's proposals—if enacted—will almost certainly do more for elementary and secondary education than any previously sent to Congress.

## THE ELEMENTARY AND SECONDARY EDUCATION ACT OF 1965: AN ANALYSIS [2]

*If we are learning anything from our experiences, we are learning that it is time for us to go to work, and the first work of these times and the first work of our society is education.*— President Lyndon B. Johnson, July 28, 1964.

Education history was written this month [April 1965] when President Johnson signed into law the Elementary and Secondary Education Act of 1965.

The purpose of the new law, which authorizes more than $1.3 billion in Federal funds to be channeled into the nation's classrooms, is to:

Strengthen elementary and secondary school programs for educationally deprived children in low income areas

Provide additional school library resources, textbooks, and other instructional materials

Finance supplementary educational centers and services

Broaden areas of cooperative research

Strengthen state departments of education

[2] From " '. . . The First Work of These Times . . .'; a Description and Analysis of the Elementary and Secondary Education Act of 1965." *American Education.* 1:13-20. Ap. '65. *American Education* is a publication of the United States Office of Education.

Actual funds still must be provided through a separate appropriations bill.

In this . . . section, *American Education* presents a description and analysis of the five titles of the new act and tells how it would be administered and financed once funds would be available.

AN ACT

To strengthen and improve educational quality and educational opportunities in the Nation's elementary and secondary schools.

TITLE I—FINANCIAL ASSISTANCE TO LOCAL EDUCATIONAL AGENCIES FOR SPECIAL EDUCATIONAL PROGRAMS IN AREAS HAVING HIGH CONCENTRATIONS OF LOW-INCOME FAMILIES

*Background:* It has long been apparent that there is a close relationship between poverty and the lack of educational development and poor academic performance. The ten states with lowest per capita personal incomes have Selective Service rejection rates for mental tests well above the average for the fifty states. Dropout rates are high where income rates are low. Economic deprivation often precludes children from taking full advantage of such educational facilities as are provided.

There is no lack of techniques, equipment, or materials which can be used or developed to meet the problem of educating the economically and culturally deprived child. But those school districts which need these materials most are least able to pay for them.

*Provisions:* This title authorizes approximately $1.06 billion to help local school districts broaden and strengthen public school programs where there are concentrations of educationally disadvantaged children. The money could be used to hire additional staff, construct facilities, acquire equipment, etc.

The amount each local school district would get would depend on two factors:

1. The average annual current expenditure per school child in the entire state

2. The number of school-age children in the district from families with annual incomes of less than $2,000 and those in families receiving more than $2,000 annually from the program of Aid to Families with Dependent Children

One half the first, multiplied by the second, would be the amount for which a local district would be eligible.

The local educational agency could use these funds as it saw fit for the benefit of deprived students of both public and nonpublic schools, through such arrangements as dual enrollment, educational media centers, and mobile educational services and equipment. Administrative supervision and control of the programs—and title to any property constructed or purchased—would rest with a public agency.

The President is required under the act to appoint a National Advisory Council on the Education of Disadvantaged Children. This Council would review the administration and operation of Title I each year, particularly the title's effectiveness in improving the educational attainment of deprived children.

*How program would work:* The Office of Education would allocate the money to state educational agencies, which have full responsibility to see that the purposes of the act are carried out. The amount each local education agency would get varies with the yardstick of poverty established by the act: the number of school-age children from low-income families. The Bureau of the Census would determine this for counties, cities, and towns where the school district is geographically identical to one of these jurisdictions.

Each local education agency must come up with its own plan for upgrading the education of deprived children and submit it to the state for approval or disapproval. The state would take into account such factors as the size of the program, its quality, and its promise of success. Local education agencies must set up evaluation procedures, such as reading tests.

*Practical application:* Needs and requirements would vary from state to state . . . and district to district. The type of programs which would best meet these needs and requirements would be left to the discretion and judgment of the state and local public educational agencies. A program effective in a rural area might be entirely inappropriate for an urban area and vice versa. A whole school system might be basically a low-income area. The best approach there might be to upgrade the regular program.

The new legislation encourages local school districts to use imaginative thinking and new approaches to meet the educational needs of deprived children. During congressional hearings on this act, witnesses testified about the following programs already being considered or conducted by educators:

In-service training for teachers

Additional teaching personnel

Teacher aides

Supervisory personnel and full-time specialists for improvement of instruction

Supplementary instructional materials

Curriculum material center for disadvantaged children

Classes for talented students

Special classes for physically handicapped, disturbed, and socially maladjusted children

Preschool training programs

Enrichment program on Saturday mornings

Programed instruction

English programs for non-English-speaking children

Special audio-visuals for disadvantaged children

Programs for the early identification of dropouts

Increased guidance services for pupils and families

School-job coordinators

Home and school visitors or social workers

Supplemental health and food services

Language laboratories, science and reading laboratories

School health, psychiatric, and psychological services

Provision of clothing, shoes, books

Financial assistance to needy high school pupils

School plant improvements—elementary school laboratories, kitchens, and cafeterias

Equip elementary classrooms for television and radio

Purchase musical recordings of classical nature, and recordings of poems and addresses

Summer school and day camp

Work experience programs

On-the-job training for high school students

Field trips for cultural and educational development

Scheduling of concerts, dramas, and lectures; mobile art exhibits and libraries

Bookmobiles to visit homes

TITLE II—SCHOOL LIBRARY RESOURCES, TEXTBOOKS, AND OTHER INSTRUCTIONAL MATERIALS

*Background:* Educational specialists—from the fields of both instruction and library science—have pointed up the growing importance of well-stocked libraries, audio-visual materials, and up-to-date textbooks and materials in an effective program of instruction.

Quality in school library programs is related to students' academic achievement, to remaining in high school, and to continuing on to college or a job. Where there are central libraries in elementary schools, research has found that children not only read more but show significant educational gains between the fourth and sixth grades. Despite this and other evidence of the value of elementary school libraries, nearly 47 per cent of public and more than 50 per cent of nonpublic elementary school students have no library. Secondary school students are somewhat better off, but the number of libraries is still inadequate. . . . Approximately 12 million of 41 million public and nonpublic elementary and secondary school students in the United States—nearly a third of them—attend schools without libraries.

The need is not confined to small school systems or to particular geographic regions. In 1963, public schools in the 21 largest U.S. cities provided fewer books per pupil and spent less per pupil than did many smaller systems which themselves had inadequate libraries.

As far as textbooks are concerned, school systems in 33 cities of over 90,000 population do not provide free high school textbooks. Nonpublic schools rarely provide free textbooks. A family with children in high school may have to spend $15 to $20 per student for up-to-date texts. In 1961, parents spent more than $90 million for textbooks—40 per cent of that year's total textbook expenditures.

*Provisions*: This title authorizes the allotment of $100 million to states for school library resources, textbooks, and other instructional materials. Materials could include books, periodicals, documents, magnetic tapes, phonograph records, and other printed and published materials. Allotments would be made on the basis of the number of children enrolled in public and nonpublic elementary and secondary schools within each state.

For the first fiscal year in which the program is in operation, up to 5 per cent of each state's grant would be available to defray administrative costs; after the first year, up to 3 per cent.

*How program would work*: The responsibility for the program would rest with the state to designate one agency to administer the state plan. In most cases this would be the state education agency. In order to participate, the state would submit to the Office of Education a plan, drafted within the framework of state laws, spelling out criteria to be used in allocating funds. The state plan would take into consideration the need of children and teachers for such materials and provide assurance that such materials would be provided on an equitable basis for all elementary and secondary school children and teachers. Materials would belong to a public agency and would be loaned—not given away.

The Federal funds for school library materials could not be substituted for state or local funds already being spent. The Federal money would have to be used to improve present programs.

The selection of all books and other instructional materials for particular schools and student bodies would be left to state and local educational authorities or agencies. States would have wide latitude in running their programs. Conceivably, a state could spend all of its allocation on library materials or textbooks.

Materials purchased with Federal funds could not be used for sectarian instruction or religious worship and when made available for the use of students in nonpublic schools would have to be the same as those used or approved for use in a state's public schools. In states legally unable to provide materials for students in nonpublic schools, the United States Commissioner of Education would make available to those children the same materials as are used in the public school. As with materials issued by states, these would be on loan.

*Practical application*: As each state must conform to its own laws, it is clear that plans regarding administration of the program would vary from state to state. In some instances the state might establish a central public depository within a school district where all school children and teachers could check out textbooks and other materials. In these cases, procedures would have to be adopted to assure the state authority an accounting of the use of the material and its proper return for reassignment.

### TITLE III—SUPPLEMENTARY EDUCATIONAL CENTERS AND SERVICES

*Background*: Among the variety of supplementary services that make the difference between a poor school and a good school are special instruction in science, languages, music, and the arts; counseling and guidance; health and social work; access to such resources as technical institutes, museums, art galleries, and theaters; and the availability of informal model innovative programs to serve as stimuli to local planning and operation.

Seventy per cent of the nation's public secondary schools have no language laboratories. Seventy-five per cent of our elementary schools do not have the services of a guidance counselor as often as once a week. In forty states, there are still secondary schools without science laboratories. Model programs have traditionally been developed only in local communities with extraordinary financial capacity and a strong commitment to education.

Many other examples of uneven distribution and inconsistent quality of educational, scientific, and cultural resources could be cited. Enrichment of the curriculum of elementary and secondary schools through supplementary services is essential.

*Provisions*: Title III authorizes $100 million for supplementary educational centers and services. The program would serve three basic functions: (1) To improve education by enabling a community to provide services not now available to the children who live there; (2) to raise the quality of educational services already offered; and (3) to stimulate and assist in the development and establishment of exemplary elementary and secondary school educational programs to serve as models for regular school programs.

A state's allocation would be based on a formula taking into account both the school-age population and the total population of the entire state. Grants, however, would be made to local public educational agencies by the Commissioner after review and recommendation by the state.

The Commissioner would have to ascertain that grants are equitably distributed according to size and population of the states, the geographic distribution of population within each state, the relative need of people in different geographic areas within the state for the kinds of services to be offered, and the relative ability of particular local educational agencies to provide these services.

The act provides that an Advisory Committee on Supplementary Educational Centers and Services be established, consisting of the Commissioner, as chairman, and eight appointed members. This committee would advise the Commissioner on action to be taken regarding applications for grants, on policy questions arising in the administration of the program, and on the development of evaluative criteria.

*How program would work*: The local educational agency or agencies applying for a grant would have to involve persons broadly representative of the cultural and educational resources of the area to help plan and carry out the local program. Such resources could include state educational agencies, colleges and universities, nonprofit private schools, libraries, museums, artistic and musical organizations, educational radio and TV, and other cultural and educational resources. The local agency's application for a grant would be based on its own perception of need and interest.

Before the Commissioner could authorize a grant, the local agency would have to meet certain criteria pertaining to fiscal responsibility, maintenance of local effort, and availability of the proposed service to all appropriate children from both public and nonprofit nonpublic schools. Its application must have been submitted to the state department of education for review and recommendation.

*Practical application*: Provision might be made for such supplementary educational services and activities as guidance and counseling, remedial instruction, school health services, vocational guidance, adult education, dual enrollment programs, and specialized instruction in advanced science, foreign languages, and other academic subjects not taught in the local schools. Cultural resources which could be drawn upon might include symphony orchestras, museums, planetariums, theaters, and the like. Special equipment and special personnel—such as artists and musicians—could be made available on a temporary basis to public and other nonprofit schools, organizations, and institutions.

Materials centers could be established to furnish modern instructional equipment and materials to area schools. A teacher might one day be in a position to call up her local center, ask for a packet of materials for a given subject at a particular grade level, and get books, films, slides, graphics, and demonstration materials the next day.

If necessary, facilities might be leased or constructed, and necessary equipment might be acquired. Mobile libraries, mobile science and language laboratories, home study courses, radio, TV, or visiting teacher programs could also be supported.

In such facilities, reasonable provision, consistent with the intended services, would have to be made for areas adaptable to artistic and cultural activities. Title to the facilities would reside in a public educational agency.

One important aspect of the program is the authorization permitting the program to aid in the development of exemplary school programs. There exists at the present time virtually no systematic institutional format for translating education research and innovation into practical innovative school programs. An important thrust of this title is to provide a means for stimulating and assisting in the development of such model demonstration programs. The hope is that many local educational agencies with the assistance they would get from Federal funds would be able to provide examples of educational innovation in practice so that teachers, administrators, and school policy planners all over the nation could observe, evaluate, and adapt these model programs to suit their own needs and purposes.

But each center or service would be tailored to the community's specific needs; designed to make optimum use of community resources. Local initiative would be used in planning, proposing, and operating the services. They would rest on a foundation of community cooperation and participation.

### TITLE IV—EDUCATIONAL RESEARCH AND TRAINING

*Background*: During this fiscal year, $34 billion is being devoted to education—which, with 26,000 operating school districts and 2,100 institutions of higher education, is America's largest industry. But only $72 million—less than one fifth of 1 per cent—is being spent on education research and development. Many private industries devote as much as 10 per cent of their annual expenditures to research and development activities.

Since 1954, the Cooperative Research Act has supported education research by colleges, universities, and state educational agencies. Such research has made significant contributions to improve students' learning. In some schools two- and three-year olds are learning to read and write. First-graders are dealing with the concepts of economics. Fourth-graders are using the set theory in mathematics. Junior high school students are studying concepts of anthropology. High school students are studying advanced science and literature courses formerly taught only in a college.

For fiscal year 1965, some $16 million was allocated under the Cooperative Research program. This is far from adequate. Moreover, even if more money was available, few colleges or state agencies have the equipment or plant to carry on extensive research and training programs.

*Provisions*: Title IV amends the Cooperative Research Act to authorize $100 million over the next five years for the construction of national and regional research facilities. In addition to the construction funds, there is authorization for an expansion of the current programs of research and development. There would also be established a new program of training for education researchers.

*How program would work*: Funds would be provided for construction and programs of national and regional laboratories. Proposals for laboratory grants would be drawn up by groups representing state departments of education, local school systems, and universities. Programs would generally be centered in areas of population concentration where an adequate operating staff may be assembled, but laboratory activities would extend throughout each region.

Four modest and necessarily incomplete forerunners of the proposed regional laboratories are now operating under the Office of Education's Research and Development Program. One in Pittsburgh is providing programs of individualized instruction based on capacity rather than age. A center at the University of Oregon is studying the structure of school-community relations and the way educational policies are formed and decisions are put into effect. At the University of Wisconsin, researchers, scholars, and teachers are working as a team on the central problems of learning—how much, how early, how quickly, and how well children can learn. A center at Harvard is concerning itself with problems presented by psychological and cultural differences among school children.

There would be no rigid formula—no magic combination of ingredients—that would have to go into every laboratory.

Needs and resources of each region would vary, and those setting up lab programs would come up with individual solutions to their individual area problems. Universities would probably play a major leadership role.

All grant proposals would be reviewed by a research advisory council. Final review would be made by the Commissioner of Education. The Office estimates that as many as eight laboratories—regionally distributed—will be planned, under construction, or built by the end of fiscal 1966.

*Practical application*: This title would both strengthen and expand the Cooperative Research Act. It would extend the authority of the Office of Education to utilize the research competence of a variety of groups and individuals heretofore excluded from participation in OE funds for research and development.

Colleges, universities, and state departments of education—which have been the sole recipients of support under the Cooperative Research program—would, of course, participate. But others would be involved. Artists, historians, mathematicians, and other scholars would work closely with psychologists, sociologists, teachers, and administrators from local school systems. They would conduct research, develop the results into forms that can be used in classrooms, continually test and retest these new forms, train teachers in their use, and make them available to local school systems.

Laboratories would provide classroom facilities where teaching experiments could be conducted and newly developed techniques might be demonstrated and evaluated. Centrally-located automatic data storage and retrieval systems might be installed—compatible systems, so that labs in other areas could exchange information. The area of teacher education would be thoroughly explored. It is conceivable that training programs could be developed to enable talented undergraduates to teach as interns in elementary and secondary schools.

TITLE V—STRENGTHENING STATE DEPARTMENTS OF EDUCATION

*Background*: If American elementary and secondary education is to be both free and effective, state departments of education must be strong. The alternative to strong state departments is an educational lag and a default of leadership.

In one medium-sized department in a middle-income state, there are 75 professional staff members. These 75 must assist 1,300 schools and 20,000 local school people in the administration of state and Federal funds and programs, in the improvement of instruction, and in the solution of technical problems relating to building, equipment, etc. Some estimate they visit each school in their state on the average of one half day every seven years. Under such circumstances—believed to be widespread—effective state educational leadership for the challenges of today and the awesome responsibilities of tomorrow is impossible.

*Provisions*: Title V authorizes $25 million for the development, improvement, or expansion of a variety of programs and projects designed to improve the effectiveness of operations of state departments of education.

For the first two years the Federal Government would bear the entire cost. Thereafter, grants would be on a matching basis, with the Federal share ranging from 50 per cent to 66 per cent.

Two types of grants are authorized: basic grants and special project grants. Eighty-five per cent of authorized funds would be for basic grants. The remainder would be for the support of experimental projects or the establishment of special services which hold promise of contributing to the solution of problems common to all or several of the states.

Provision is made for an interchange of personnel between the Office of Education and state educational agencies. The commissioner of Education might arrange for assignments of Office of Education personnel to state departments, or state personnel to the Office of Education, for a period not exceeding two years.

An Advisory Council on State Departments of Education is to be appointed by the Secretary of Health, Education, and Welfare. This council would review the administration of programs for which Federal funds are appropriated, not only under this title, but under all other acts which provide funds to assist state education agencies in administering Federal programs in education.

*How program would work*: State departments, when applying for grants, would review their present programs, indicating where their needs are greatest.

Funds could be used to improve educational planning; identify educational problems and needs; evaluate educational programs; record, collect, process, analyze, interpret, store, retrieve, and report educational data; publish and distribute curriculum materials; conduct educational research; improve teacher preparation; train individuals to serve state and local educational agencies; and provide consultative and technical assistance in special areas of educational need.

## CIVIL RIGHTS ENFORCEMENT [3]

Perhaps no single event engendered as much optimism over the prospects for eradicating racial discrimination in public education as enactment of the Civil Rights Act of 1964. Much of this optimism was based upon Title VI of the act, which provides in Section 601 that "No person in the United States shall, on grounds of race, color, or national origin, be excluded from participation in, be denied the benefits of, or be subjected to discrimination under any program or activity receiving Federal financial assistance."

The enforcement of Section 601 is especially important to public education. Federal spending for education has increased from $4,650 million in 1964 to $6,328 million in 1965, and is expected to reach $8,711 million in 1966, almost 8 per cent of the total revenues for public elementary and secondary schools. The dollar amounts are only part of the picture. The major Federal appropriations for public schools flow from the Elementary and Secondary Education Act of 1965. The Johnson Administration avoided both the racial and religious issues which had previously held up large-scale Federal aid by emphasizing aid to children from low-income families, i.e., families with an income of $2,000 or less and from families on ADC [Aid to Dependent Children]. This approach made excellent educational as well as political sense, since the educational disabilities of such children are a more urgent problem than the acknowledged need to improve the education of middle- and upper-class children. However, although the formula for allocating aid under the Elementary and Secondary Education Act is geared to the number of low-income families in states and school districts, the act includes virtually no safeguards to insure that the funds appropriated are effectively—or even actually—used for the education of children from such families. In effect, the act provides for general aid to education distributed to school districts according to the number of children from low-income families in such districts.

[3] From "The Civil Rights Fiasco in Public Education," by Myron Lieberman, director of educational research and development, Rhode Island College, and former consultant to the National Association for the Advancement of Colored People. *Phi Delta Kappan.* 47:482-6. My. '66. Reprinted by permission. Text from reprint in *Teachers College Record.* 68:120-6. N. '66.

In 1963, the median income of Negroes was only 53 per cent of that for the white population. Obviously, large-scale Federal aid for the education of children from low-income families will be of enormous assistance to Negro children if such aid is used in a non-discriminatory way. The sad truth is, however, that despite Section 601 the administration of Federal aid to education, including aid for the education of children from low-income families, is frequently characterized by blatant discrimination against Negro students. Quite often, such discrimination is most widespread and most repressive precisely in the communities where there is greatest need to upgrade the education of Negro children. Over-all, the extent of discrimination varies from school system to school system and its extent is somewhat imprecise, but it is clearly very substantial. The purpose of this article is to explain why this is so and to suggest some steps which might improve the situation.

## The Uses of Title VI

Under Title VI, each Federal department and agency extending financial assistance was directed to issue, subject to presidential approval, whatever regulations were needed to implement Section 601. The regulations concerning HEW [Department of Health, Education, and Welfare] programs were approved by the President on December 3, 1964. They provided that a school system would be deemed in compliance if (1) it gave assurance of compliance with a final order of a United States court for desegration of the system; or (2) it submitted a desegregation plan acceptable to the Commissioner of Education and assurances that the system would implement the plan.

Subsequently, several school systems submitted compliance plans which United States Commissioner of Education Francis Keppel deemed unacceptable. As a result, Keppel came under increasing pressure to formulate a more specific set of guidelines for school systems seeking compliance. Finally, on April 29, 1965, after considerable discussion and controversy between and within a number of Federal agencies, Keppel issued a *General Statement of Policies Under Title VI of the Civil Rights Act of 1964 Respect-*

*ing Desegregation of Elementary and Secondary Schools,* now universally known as "the Guidelines." A revised version of the Guidelines was issued on March 7, 1966. To a large extent, the effectiveness of Section 601 in public education depends upon the nature of the obligations to desegregate imposed by the Guidelines and the extent to which these obligations are enforced. It is important, therefore, to consider these matters carefully.

The 1965 Guidelines provided three methods of compliance with Title VI. One was by executing HEW Form 441, an Assurance of Compliance. However, school systems characterized by "any . . . practices characteristic of dual or segregated systems" were prohibited from executing an Assurance of Compliance. An Assurance of Compliance was supposed to be executed only by school systems in which segregation in any form is not a problem.

School systems subject to a final order of a United States court to desegregate the entire system were also to be regarded as in compliance, provided that the systems promised to comply with the court order and any future modifications. Finally, school systems still characterized by segregation in some form but not under a final court order to desegregate (the category into which most southern school systems fall) were required to submit a desegregation plan which the Commissioner deemed adequate to accomplish the purposes of the Civil Rights Act. The Guidelines required such plans to meet nonracial criteria for zoning; assignment; reassignment; transfer; faculty; and availability of services, facilities, and programs. School systems submitting desegregation plans had to desegregate at least four grades beginning in the 1965-66 school year, and the fall of 1967 had to be accepted as the target date for complete desegregation. Throughout this period, the school systems were to submit compliance reports concerning such matters as the racial distribution of children and staff in schools and attendance zones; the rules for assignment, reassignment, and transfer; and the status of any legal proceedings relating to desegregation.

### Guidelines Relatively Ineffective

By the summer of 1965, it was evident that the Guidelines were not going to effectuate compliance with Section 601 in hundreds of school systems. This ineffectiveness was publicly conceded by United States Commissioner of Education Harold Howe II. In announcing revision of the Guidelines on March 7, 1966, Howe pointed out that about 180,000 Negro children were attending schools also attended by white children in the eleven Deep South states. This figure represented less than 6 per cent of the total number of Negro children in these states. As Howe pointed out, the Guidelines did not deal with discrimination in school systems which had not formally operated segregated school systems. Although he did not mention the enormous discrimination prevailing even in systems where some desegregation resulted from the Guidelines, Howe stated that "This year, the emphasis will be shifted from negotiation to performance" and that "Summing up, we are now concluding what some have called the 'paper compliance' phase of our Title VI operations."

In practice, the 1965 Guidelines did not bring about a substantial degree of compliance with Section 601. Strategies of evasion were—and are—based upon local conditions. Where there is a high degree of residential segregation, school boards have adopted strict geographical zones. Despite a specific HEW regulation prohibiting site selection to maximize segregation, new schools—often unnecessary ones if existing capacity were utilized on a nonracial basis—are being located to do just that. Indeed, one of the most disturbing aspects of the present situation is the lack of opposition to the frantic southern drive to build new schools where they will maximize segregation for many years to come.

Actually, there is far less residential segregation in large southern cities than in large northern communities. Thus most large southern communities seeking to avoid desegregation do so by adopting "freedom of choice" plans. Under these plans, pupils may elect to attend any school in the district which has space for them. The Guidelines permit such plans despite the fact that they are usually adopted to bring about indirectly what Title VI forbids school systems to accomplish directly. According to the Guidelines, however, such plans must provide adequate opportunity to make a choice, ample notice of procedures for initial assignment, preregistration, enrollment, reassignment, transfer, assignment on a nonracial basis in cases of overcrowding, availability of transportation on a nonracial basis, and assurances that school personnel will not favor or penalize pupils for the choices they make.

During 1965-66, freedom of choice plans typically resulted in complete segregation or tokenism. Notice to Negro parents and students was minimal. The administrative procedures which had to be followed to challenge a school board action were typically designed to place the protester at an overwhelming disadvantage. For example, in Jefferson County, Alabama, parents who challenged the school board assignment had to apply for a transfer in person to an all-white agency in a segregated county office building. The school administration could postpone the required hearing at will without notice, but a parent failure to attend was deemed withdrawal of the application for transfer. Failure of the pupil to appear at any hearing, examination, or test required could also be deemed withdrawal of the application.

In many school districts, Negroes who enroll their children in white schools are subject to severe economic and physical coercion. Such coercion might be less effective if large numbers of Negroes enrolled in white schools, but this seldom happens. Thus heavy pressure on a small activist minority usually suffices to maintain tokenism or even complete segregation, e.g., the Jefferson County system, with 45,000 white and 18,000 Negro pupils, had not a single white or Negro student attending school with students of the other race from the initiation of its transfer plan in January, 1959, to the summer of 1965.

Freedom of choice plans would be less discriminatory if there were desegregation of teachers within school systems adopting such plans. In fact, the ramifications of teacher employment for Section 601 are much broader than is generally understood and required some elaboration. As long as schools are staffed on a segregated basis, it will be extremely difficult to achieve desegregation at the pupil level. The white community inevitably regards the white-teacher school as "our" school and seeks to transfer white pupils to it. Schools staffed entirely by Negro teachers are just as inevitably regarded as Negro schools, to which all Negro pupils must be directed.

Many communities operate low-enrollment schools which should be closed. In situations where the Negro school is closed, a common practice is to release all the Negro teachers on the ground that their jobs no longer exist. In many cases, experienced Negro teachers are released, while beginning white teachers are employed in the consolidated school or in the school system. The situation is analogous to the industrial issue of plant- or company-wide seniority. When a Negro school is discontinued, teacher tenure tends to be based upon seniority in the school being discontinued, not in the school system as a whole. The upshot is the dismissal of experienced Negro teachers simultaneously with the employment of new white teachers.

In many Negro communities, Negro teachers occupy important leadership positions. These teachers, and the Negro community generally, face a cruel dilemma when school boards threaten—unofficially but nonetheless unmistakably—to fire as many Negro teachers as possible if Negro children apply to white schools under a freedom of choice plan. In some districts, teacher contracts are held up until the deadline for Negro pupils to apply for transfer to white schools. Negro parents find it difficult to press for such transfers when they are likely to result in the wholesale dismissal of Negro teachers.

## Guidelines Revised

How will the preceding problems be affected by the 1966 Guidelines? Clearly, the 1966 Guidelines provide a better basis for coping with them than the 1965 version did. For example, the 1965 Guidelines required only that "Steps shall also be taken toward the elimination of segregation of teaching and staff personnel in the schools resulting from prior assignments based on race, color, or national origin." By contrast, the 1966 Guidelines require "significant progress beyond what was accomplished for the 1965-66 school year in the desegregation of teachers assigned to schools on a regular full-time basis." This provision is especially important, because the revised Guidelines also require school authorities to close "small inadequate schools that were originally established for students of a particular race and are still used primarily or exclusively for the education of students of such race . . . if the facilities, teaching materials, or educational programs available to students in such a school are inferior to those generally available in the schools of the system." It is therefore likely that discrimination against Negro teachers will be an even greater problem during 1966 than it has been in the past. This means that unless the 1966 Guidelines are enforced effectively, thousands of Negro teachers and administrators are likely to be dismissed, downgraded, or not employed solely on a racial basis during the year. Under the 1966 Guidelines, a student must be given freedom of choice every year and the administration of freedom of choice plans includes a number of safeguards not present in the earlier Guidelines. The texts for the letter, explanatory notice, and freedom of choice plan to be sent to parents are prescribed by the Commissioner of Education. Parents and students may, however, indicate their choice of school in writing on other forms, and, so long as they are clear, such preferences may not be disregarded by school authorities. Choices may not be changed except under specified conditions, a safeguard designed to prevent coercion against Negro parents and children to change their choices. Choices must be honored unless overcrowding results, in which case students must be assigned on the basis of proximity to the school. Information concerning choices by individuals is not to be made public by the school system, and there are other provisions designed to ensure that freedom of choice plans cannot be used to block desegregation as they have in the past.

Despite these improvements in the Guidelines, widespread violation of Section 601 is likely to prevail for many years. The Guidelines must be enforced, and despite much brave talk, enforcement is minimal. Officially, enforcement is a staff responsibility of David Seeley, who heads USOE's [United States Office of Education] Office of Equal Educational Opportunity. Seeley's good faith and dedication are widely accepted, but the crucial decisions and policies concerning enforcement are made at cabinet and presidential levels. At these levels, vigorous enforcement endangers other political objectives. Furthermore, the Office of Education, like so many other Federal agencies, is extremely sensitive to congressional pressures, and congressmen are far more likely to protest vigorous enforcement than they are to protest the absence of it. When a congressman protests an act of enforcement, he usually does so on direct request of his constituents; the congressman who protects weak enforcement usually does so on behalf of persons outside his constituency, hence his involvement is not likely to be as urgent. Furthermore, the opposition to enforcement is not entirely from the South; if it were, enforcement would be much more vigorous.

Enforcement problems are different for new programs which do not require periodic allocations than for programs already under way. Technically, the Commissioner of Education need not terminate assistance in the first situation even if he believes there is noncompliance. He need only . . . refuse to authorize assistance. Since administrative agencies are accorded a reasonable time to act and there is no deadline they have to meet, the Commissioner is in a relatively strong negotiating position in this situation.

With programs already under way, the Commissioner must terminate assistance if he cannot bring about compliance. The termination must be preceded by "an express finding on the record, after opportunity for hearing, of a failure to comply." Furthermore, the Commissioner must file a full written report of the circumstances and grounds for action with appropriate House and Senate committees, and no termination is to be effective until thirty days after the filing of these reports. The difficulty of securing compliance under this procedure is dramatized by the fact that it was not until March 31, 1966, that the Office of Education mailed its first official notice of a hearing to a school system charged with failure to live up to a desegregation plan previously accepted as compliance with the Guidelines. This notice was mailed to school authorities in Baker County, Georgia, where a USOE reporting team found flagrant violations of the plan and recommended an immediate cutoff of Federal funds in September, 1965. In fact, the school authorities conceded in September, 1965, that they were not in compliance, yet they have received Federal funds throughout the 1965-66 school year and will continue to do so this spring regardless of the outcome of the hearing.

## USOE Limitations

The notice to the Baker County school system received widespread publicity, but most southern school officials have already seen that the USOE's bark is worse than its bite. Actually, the USOE compliance staff is much too small to cope with the legal and administrative problems posed by the withholding provisions of the Civil Rights Act. In early March of 1966, only 53 of the 103 authorized professional positions on the compliance staff were filled, yet there seemed to be little sense of urgency in filling the vacant positions.

The problems of enforcing compliance are also compounded by the requirement in the Civil Rights Act that limits withholding of Federal funds to the particular program in the particular political entity, or part thereof, in which noncompliance is found. Thus if a community gives white pupils preferential treatment in the distribution of equipment purchased under the National Defense Education Act, and if this were established according to the procedures set forth in Title VI, the withholding of Federal funds would nevertheless be limited to this particular program.

The limitation of withholding to the particular political entity concerned also raises some difficult questions. The Clarksdale, Mississippi, School Board is under a court order to desegregate its first two grades. Pursuant to this order, the board drew new attendance zones which included white and Negro pupils. Rather, it included them until the Negro homes were torn down or physically moved to another part of the city as part of an urban renewal program. The urban renewal program was allegedly never discussed with the school board, but it played a key role in keeping the schools segregated. Another cluster of Negro homes near a white school was disannexed by the city, thereby forcing the Negro pupils living in these homes to attend a segregated county school for Negroes. In short, Title VI is inadequate to end discrimination by political entities which act to perpetuate segregation in programs supported by Federal funds but which do not themselves receive such funds.

One hopeful development is that, although the Guidelines are criticized for accepting judicial timetables for desegregation, they have already been cited by some courts as a basis for speeding up these timetables. On this score, a June 21, 1965, decision by the Fifth Circuit Federal Court in *Singleton* vs. *Jackson* [Mississippi] *Municipal Separate School District* may presage a basic change in judicial opinion. In the Singleton case, the Negro plaintiffs sued to enjoin the Jackson board from proceeding with a grade-a-year plan that had failed to proceed even this slowly. In upholding the injunction, Judge John Minor Wisdom stated that the board should desegregate at least as rapidly as it would have been required to do by the Guidelines. He asserted that judges, who are not educational experts, should not delay desegregation more than administrative agencies set up to rule on these matters. Wisdom also indicated that the court would rely heavily upon the Guidelines and would not reward intransigent school systems by allowing them more time to desegregate than the Guidelines do. Indeed, his opinion went far toward discarding the entire notion of "all deliberate speed" as a prolonged deprivation of the constitutional rights of the Negro plaintiffs.

If widely followed, Wisdom's opinion could have a profound effect upon future developments. Since 1954, the courts have had to grapple with timetables for desegregation without help or guidance from any authoritative educational agency. Instead, the administrative agencies have looked to the courts for guidance. The Singleton case reverses this emphasis. The courts now have a standard which will enable them to get out of the school board business. If they do so by relying upon the Guidelines, desegregation may be speeded up on a broad front.

## The Need for Speed

Title VI is not self-enforcing and local action on a broad scale will be essential to implement it. For this reason, Title VI will result in more, not fewer, protests against discrimination. It may also result in more desegregation by the fall of 1966 than took place between 1954 and 1964. This prediction by its more optimistic supporters is probably accurate, but it tells more about the slow pace of desegregation than the long-range benefits of Title VI. For over a decade, efforts to get a few Negro children in white schools have absorbed a considerable share of the resources of the civil rights movement. The need is for faster progress at the policy-making levels—legislatures, state departments of education, school boards, boards of trustees, and so on. Without effective support for desegregation at these levels, tokenism is likely to prevail for many years to come. One need not derogate tokenism to see this; tokenism may be a necessary point of achievement and departure on the road to full desegregation. Still, it is unfortunate that Section 601 and the Guidelines are focused almost exclusively at the pupil and teacher level while discrimination in the policy-making and administrative echelons of public education are hardly mentioned. At best, Section 601 is essentially a tool whose efficacy will depend in large measure upon when, where, how, and by whom it is wielded. To this observer, indications are that it is being wielded too little and too late to achieve the goal for which it was enacted.

## FEDERAL PRESSURES ON THE NORTH [4]

Federal programs to help "desegregate" schools in northern cities have run into a challenge in Congress.

The challenge came on August 23 from Representative William C. Cramer (Republican), of Florida.

Representative Cramer charged that the United States Office of Education "appears to be violating" the 1964 Civil Rights Act by granting more than $730,000 of Federal funds "to implement experiments attacking de facto segregation or racial imbalance" in northern schools.

Mr. Cramer wrote the United States Commissioner of Education, Harold Howe II, asking "under what authority" his office is making such grants and told the House, "I intend to pursue this matter."

[4] From "Is Federal Aid Helping to End Neighborhood Schools?" *U.S. News & World Report.* 61:49-50. S. 5, '66. Reprinted from *U.S. News & World Report*, published at Washington.

Mr. Howe, on August 25, denied Mr. Cramer's charge and said "a full, responsive reply to the Congressman's inquiry is being prepared."

The issue raised in this dispute is one that could decide the fate of the system of "neighborhood schools" that is used in the North. That issue:

Is there any legal authority for Federal action to break up the kind of "segregation" found in the North?

This so-called de facto segregation is not caused by the exclusion of Negroes from white schools. It results from housing patterns, with Negroes concentrated in neighborhoods that are nearly all-Negro, and with children attending schools in their neighborhoods.

The Supreme Court has never held that this is unconstitutional.

Congress has tried to exclude de facto segregation as a target of its civil rights legislation.

Mr. Howe complained recently that in trying to attack the northern style of "segregation," Federal officials run into "quicksands of legal interpretation." He said: "We can't do anything; we can only suggest and stimulate local school districts."

Many Federal officials, however, have come out with "suggestions"—and Federal "stimulation" is being given to a variety of local actions.

Much of the "stimulation" to local action has come in the form of Federal money. Some of this money has come from funds appropriated for aid for education—not from the civil rights funds cited by Representative Cramer.

East Orange, New Jersey, for example, has received $162,000 of Federal aid-to-education money for planning an "educational plaza" which would serve to bring together school facilities now scattered widely around the city.

The East Orange idea is to "phase out all neighborhood schools" and replace them with a central complex that would provide "a common educational experience for children and youth from all sections of the city—rich and poor, Negro and white."

East Orange officials are hoping for additional Federal funds in carrying out this plan.

## Other Cities, Other Methods

Similar ideas for central "educational parks" or "plazas" are being discussed in several cities.

Mt. Vernon, New York, is counting on Federal assistance to establish a model "children's academy"—using the newest educational methods—located on the fringes of white and Negro neighborhoods to attract children of both races.

This idea is in line with a recent Howe suggestion that "we will have to reappraise where the boundary lines of neighborhoods should be drawn when we speak of 'the neighborhood school.'"

Mr. Howe also suggested that the nation needs to take a "close look" at the whole system of neighborhood schools in the light of its frequent effect of separating Negroes from whites in the schoolroom.

Another Howe suggestion is that white suburbs should share the racial problems of city schools. One of his ideas is that city school districts might combine with suburban districts.

This idea has been under consideration in Atlanta, Georgia, where school authorities talk of creating a Metropolitan Educational Authority that would include the predominantly white suburbs along with the heavily Negro city.

One problem that Atlanta has encountered is that many suburban residents do not relish the idea of unification with the city.

Last May, voters of suburban Sandy Springs turned down by a vote of more than 2 to 1 a proposed annexation with Atlanta. One reason given by a Sandy Springs leader was fear "the Federal Government might compel busing of students" because "we don't have enough Negroes in our community."

Norman F. Lent, a state senator from a suburb of New York City, was quoted by the *Wall Street Journal* recently as predicting that "the time is coming when the City of New York will attempt to exchange students on a forced basis with its suburbs."

To this, according to the *Journal*, Mayor John L. Messina of suburban Port Chester replied: "Never."

Commissioner Howe warned educators in a recent speech that they must be prepared to risk "enraging suburban taxpayers" to carry out the task of desegregating northern schools.

Busing of city Negroes to suburban schools already is being tried on a small scale in several cities.

One of the Federal grants attacked by Representative Cramer gives $130,000 to a Hartford, Connecticut, experiment in which 266 pupils from heavily Negro schools in the city are to be bused into white suburbs.

This grant was made under Title IV of the 1964 Civil Rights Act, which authorizes Federal aid for dealing with problems of "desegregation."

The Federal money is not used to finance the actual busing of Hartford pupils. Instead, it goes for the pay and training of special teachers and consultants, and for "evaluation" of the results of the experiment.

Mr. Howe describes this as helping "school personnel to deal effectively with special educational problems occasioned by desegregation, which is in the authorizing language of Title IV." He insists:

"No Title IV funds are being used for transporting pupils or overcoming racial imbalance."

## A Definition of Desegregation

Mr. Cramer's position is that the Hartford grant is "part and parcel" of a program based on busing and thus "encourages what the Congress specifically forbade." He told the House:

In passing the 1964 Civil Rights Act, this body adopted my amendment to the definition of "desegregation" which says that "desegregation shall not mean the assignment of students to public schools in order to overcome racial imbalance."

In the light of this definition, Mr. Cramer said:

It becomes crystal clear that the award of Federal funds to any school board for the purpose of implementing programs aimed at overcoming de facto segregation or racial imbalance is absolutely improper. . . .

Grants are being made to northern school boards, including Hartford, Connecticut, where there has not been any deliberate segregation of students in the public schools. The only logical conclusion is that the grants are being made to overcome de facto segregation or racial imbalance.

In addition to the Hartford grant, officials of the United States Office of Education list these other grants that have been made under the Civil Rights Act for "desegregation" purposes to school systems that are outside the South:

> Los Angeles, $109,103 to train personnel in problems of desegregation
>
> New York City, $199,951 for training personnel, with one aim described as: "to develop skills in the area of civil liberties and civil rights"
>
> Oakland, California, $30,000 for "advisory specialists in solving the problems of racially and ethnically mixed schools"
>
> California state department of education, $153,901 "for a statewide advisory service for local school districts to assist them in dealing with problems incident to desegregation"
>
> New York state department of education, $85,400 "to establish a model state program for desegregation" and $8,600 for a teacher institute "on individualizing instruction for classroom integration" in two schools of New York City
>
> Syracuse, New York, $12,604 for planning a school-desegregation program

Together with the Hartford project, these grants add up to the $730,000 figure cited by Mr. Cramer.

Whatever the outcome of the Cramer challenge to such spending, the role of the Federal Government in the war on de facto segregation seems sure to grow.

Studies of northern schools are being made by the United States Civil Rights Commission and the Office of Education. Bills are pending in Congress to authorize specifically the use of Federal aid against racial imbalance.

Schools of the South have been under Federal pressure ever since the Supreme Court outlawed separate schools for Negroes in 1954. Now the pressure is shifting to the North, as well.

# IV. SOME RECENT INNOVATIONS

## EDITOR'S INTRODUCTION

With the Federal Government pouring some $9 billion a year into local school districts across the country, the wherewithal for a wide variety of innovations is now at hand. Some school districts, of course, are breaking new ground on their own. But many of the most highly publicized projects—Head Start, for example—are federally supported.

A glance at the bibliography at the end of this compilation will give the reader an inkling of the sweeping extent of the many experiments and innovations currently underway. In this section, however, we are limiting ourselves to a survey of five of the more important or interesting ones.

The first article describes an "interdisciplinary" program at De Anza High School in California, aimed at making vocational education something more than the cabinetmaking, metalworking drudgery it has been in the past. The second article describes a problem that has long nettled educators and one school district's attempt to solve it: Why must children of obviously differing capacities nonetheless climb grade by grade up an educational ladder geared more to biological than intellectual progression? In the nongraded schools of Appleton, Wisconsin, educators are experimenting—apparently with considerable success—in a more logical approach to educational advancement.

In recent months Project Head Start, which roused great hopes when first implemented, has been criticized for losing its impact on disadvantaged children once they sink back into their poverty environment. The third article gives an assessment of the Head Start program as it has developed and suggests ways in which its impact and the initial advantage it brings to the underprivileged can be maintained.

The last two articles describe innovations that are making big, one-campus schools and summer schools new forces for betterment in the learning process.

## VOCATIONAL EDUCATION: A NEW APPROACH [1]

The vast majority of our high school students are being given courses that are likely to be meaningless to them in later life. The result is a tragic waste of human potential. But now a remarkable new curriculum in California shows how to make the same courses come to life.

Let's visit a classroom in the De Anza High School in Richmond, California, across the bay from San Francisco. As you sit at the rear of the room listening to what's going on, you notice nothing unusual. The teacher is lecturing on sound waves, and it could be any physics class in the country: thirty students at their desks facing a blackboard full of wavy lines and a table loaded with complicated electronic equipment that fills the classroom with growls and shrieks.

But this is no conventional class. It is part of what's called an "interdisciplinary" approach to education, and it is being watched with growing interest by educators all over the country. For what is going on in this classroom may become the basis of the most significant of all the changes that are now transforming our educational system.

Its significance is this: Unlike the vast majority of our high school courses, this one is specifically designed to meet the needs of the students who will probably *not* go on to complete a four-year college course. Behind this aim lies a startling fact: A huge 80 per cent of the students who enter high school do not continue their education through college. Yet the basic curriculums of our school system—the "prestige" courses into which most students are forced—are dictated by the specialized needs of the 20 per cent who will go to college. The De Anza course is one of several aimed at correcting this imbalance. To appreciate what's involved, first look at the enormous waste of the present system.

[1] From "The Coming Revolution Against Boredom in the Classroom," by James Nathan Miller, a free-lance writer reporting frequently on developments in education. *PTA Magazine.* 60:18-21. Ap. '66. Reprinted with permission from *The PTA Magazine* (April 1966). Copyright 1966 by The Reader's Digest Assn., Inc. Condensed in *The Reader's Digest* (May 1966).

## *Making Education Relevant*

There are two main routes that today's student can follow through the school system—the "high road" of academic courses and the "low road" of vocational education. But regardless of which road they take, most of them run into the same trap: boredom with courses that they consider to be—and that too often are—useless.

Of those taking academic courses, for instance, about a third quit school before graduation. They just can't see the applicability of their college-oriented courses—medieval history, Chaucer, physics—to their own lives. Says Ken T. Bement, president of the Canadian subsidiary of the Burroughs Corporation, "To my mind, the high school dropout is often right—tragically right—in his evaluation of the school's potential to prepare him for the next half century of his working life." Secretary of Labor W. Willard Wirtz calls such students "pushouts."

What about those who stick it out and get a diploma? Only about half get into college, and of these roughly 40 per cent drop out in their freshman year—then go into the armed forces or the labor market, equipped with little but a fast-vanishing recollection of some chemistry formulas, a few quotes from *Macbeth,* and perhaps a smattering of typing or accounting.

What, then, about vocational education? Isn't *it* giving realistic preparation for the world of work? The answer is no, and there are two main reasons:

First, in the words of Grant Venn, author of *Man, Education and Work,* vocational education's students "too often are the dropouts or castoffs of the academic curriculum. Its teachers . . . enjoy relatively low status within the teaching profession." Vocational education, says former Ford Foundation President Henry Heald, is "the stepchild of the American education system."

Second, too often vocational courses do not teach the skills that modern industry wants. "If you visit almost any vocational school," says Edward T. Chase, a leading expert on automation and youth unemployment, "you will find its program incredibly irrelevant to the facts of work in the 1960's. [See "The Waste of Manpower,"

by Edward T. Chase, in Section II, above.] There are courses in
New York City, for instance, that teach cabinetmaking, though
there is no demand in the area for cabinetmakers.

Thus our high-road, low-road educational system is providing
a large number of students with courses that bore them. And in
our failure to motivate these students to study, we are helping to
make them useless—to themselves and to the economy. Says
Edward Chase, "The biggest failure of American education is the
way it is turning millions of young people into unemployables."

### *Experiment in California*

Which brings us back to the "interdisciplinary" classroom at
De Anza High in California. It is part of a new plan that began
in 1961 as an experiment in two Richmond, California, schools
and has since been adopted by thirteen others in the San Francisco
area.

The plan's enormous significance is stated by Massachusetts
Institute of Technology Professor N. H. Frank, former head of
MIT's physics department and now a leader in the movement to
reform vocational education. "The Richmond plan," Professor
Frank told me, "is a most hopeful start toward motivating the un-
motivated student."

It does it two ways: First, it gives the student a reason that he
can understand for studying, and then it arranges his curriculum
so that this reason runs through all his courses. Two main depar-
tures from conventional teaching are involved.

The first departure is revealed in the title of the course, "Pretechnical." What this means is that the course does not pretend
either that it's aiming its students along the high road toward a
four-year college or that it's trying to steer them to the low road
of commitment to a specific skill. It gives them a *middle* road—
preparation for further training in the vast and expanding field of
technology and perhaps, later on, transfer to a four-year college.

"This program," says one teacher, "is all carrot and no stick."
And the carrot—the field of technology—is no vague, ivory-tower
goal for the students to aim at. They can *see* what the aim is

merely by reading the Help Wanted columns of the newspapers. These include, of course, appeals for graduate engineers and Ph.D.'s, but there are hundreds more for jobs that the students can easily see are attainable for *them*.

Arde Engineering, for instance, wanted twenty-five technical illustrators. IBM had a long list of jobs immediately available for technicians to repair automated equipment, rebuild vacuum furnaces, and test electronic circuits. Emerson Radio wanted TV servicemen. National Cash Register offered to train qualified high school graduates to service its office equipment. Johnson and Hoffman Manufacturing was looking for tool- and die-makers.

All over the country students can read such ads, appealing for precisely the skills they are developing in the classroom.

Second, the Richmond plan introduces a basic change in teaching technique—interdisciplinary classes. Let's return to the De Anza classroom and listen closely. After a few minutes you'll suddenly make a surprising discovery. Despite all the electronic sound-wave paraphernalia and the scientific jottings on the blackboard, this is not a physics class. It is English.

The discussion of sound waves started with questions about pronunciation and phonetics that had grown out of the reading aloud of a student's theme. Now with equipment borrowed from the physics laboratory, the lessons in grammar, spelling, and creative writing are all linked to reports the students are doing on sound waves.

But the sound-wave discussion doesn't stop with the English class. When the students go on to the physics classroom they will continue the inquiry on a more technical level. And in math their teacher will build his lessons around the formulas that explain the workings of the sound waves. In shop the students will experiment with making the electronic circuits that produce the beeps and groans, and back in English class, other assignments will similarly plug in to the sound-wave discussions.

## Some Promising Results

How successful has the Richmond plan been? Since it has so far been operating on a pilot-project basis—sixty students a year at each of the nineteen schools—the plan's success to date must be measured by the potential it indicates rather than the statistics it has accumulated. The size of this potential is shown in what people tell me about their experiences with the Richmond plan.

Said Mrs. Jackson Chance, executive director of the Rosenberg Foundation of San Francisco: "The stir that the Richmond plan has caused in educational circles has made it one of the most significant grants we have ever made." (The Cogswell Polytechnical College of San Francisco directed the development of the new curriculum; and the Rosenberg Foundation of San Francisco and the Ford Foundation provided financial support.)

Last autumn school systems in Oregon, Michigan, and North Carolina began Richmond plan courses. More important, a study group of top educators that met last summer at MIT to consider the problems of vocational education recently announced its recommendation to the United States Office of Education: expansion of the interdisciplinary concept throughout the United States school system.

The Richmond plan has already begun to move into areas other than pretechnical. One remarkable program now being offered at six high schools in the Greater Bay area of San Francisco is called Project FEAST (Foods Education and Service Technology). This one aims at preparation for jobs in the fast-growing "hospitality" field of hotels and restaurants.

The students use the regular comprehensive faculty. But there is the same interdisciplinary technique of teaching as at De Anza. Students learn mathematics, for instance, by drawing up mass-order food purchases, figuring recipe proportions, calculating percentages of waste. English lessons are based partially on readings in hotel and restaurant trade journals.

The results? Last year, of the twenty-four students who started FEAST at the Pacific High School in San Leandro, California, twenty-two finished. This year the waiting list was so long that the faculty admitted twenty-eight students—four more than there was room for—on the assumption that five or six would drop out. But four months after the school started, it still had twenty-eight students, and no one showed signs of quitting.

Consider Rich Snyder, seventeen, a senior at Pacific High School in San Leandro:

Before this, I had no plan for the future. I was tired of school and was just taking useless courses like woodshop and metalworking. Now that I know the job I am heading for, my marks have gone 'way up, and I even have a chance for a scholarship at San Francisco State College.

And Mrs. Opal Massey, a Richmond plan teacher at Oakland Technical High School, says: "I have been in this school twenty years, and this is the first time I have felt that I am really teaching something."

A. Winston Richards, Pacific High principal, looks to the future: "Now our aim is to find other job-preparation fields to extend the plan to." Two rapidly growing job areas into which it will probably soon be extended are the automobile-servicing business and the "paramedical" field of nursing aides and technicians.

## Eliminating Boredom

Could such an approach work in your school? Only if it is adopted with the full realization that this is no mere surface rearranging of classes. The Richmond plan involves a complete revision of educational thinking. For one thing, it requires exceptional teachers. Here is the biggest problem any school will face. "Only teachers who can *bend* can work within the plan," says James Kelly, De Anza science teacher. For many, such bending is impossible; it violates most of what they learned at teachers' college and have been practicing for years in the classroom.

Some schools also will have to battle with the parents. Many push students beyond their abilities, because to many a college degree is *the* supreme status symbol. Since the Richmond plan steers students not toward a bachelor's degree but toward future training in a junior college or technical school—or, in the case of FEAST, even employment on graduation—some of the Richmond schools using the plan have met strong opposition. Others have not. It depends mainly on the kind of community the school is in.

A third problem is that such a program costs from 5 to 15 per cent more than the standard curriculum because it demands more of teachers, and teacher time is the biggest single cost in our educational system. Not only must the teachers meet several times each week to coordinate the pacing and the subject matter of their courses; they also must go to summer workshops to prepare for the new approach, and many must follow this up with long additional hours of "going back to high school" to bone up on each other's subjects.

Says Edith Hutcheson, English teacher at Oakland Technical High School:

> We've changed the vocabulary and spelling in my class so that now they're largely made up of technical and scientific words, and *I* have to know what they mean. It's taken a lot of study to learn how a viscometer works, or a planimeter, or the mathematical difference between accuracy and precision, or what "standard deviation" means.

Thus this remarkable new kind of course has ramifications that will reach deep into our educational system, affecting teachers, parents, school administrations—even teacher-training and college admission requirements. But the challenges that the Richmond plan presents, big as they are, seem small compared with the enormous hope that they hold out to the forgotten 80 per cent of our students: the hope that this middle road will free them from the biggest and most destructive trap in our educational system—boredom in the classroom.


## SCHOOLS WITHOUT GRADES [2]

There are no first, second, third, fourth, fifth or sixth grade pupils in the elementary schools of Appleton, Wisconsin. Children are ungraded. They are neither promoted nor failed. They do not receive report cards.

[2] From *Schools of Tomorrow—Today!* by Arthur D. Morse, a staff producer for CBS-TV on the CBS Reports series. Doubleday. Garden City, N.Y. '60. p 29-40. Copyright © 1960 by Arthur D. Morse. Reprinted by permission of the author and Doubleday & Company, Inc.

Under Appleton's Continuous Progress Plan, youngsters move along as fast as their individual abilities can take them. Free from the artificial limits of grade requirements they push on beyond these arbitrary boundaries. In the process they meet the toughest competitive challenge in the world—the challenge to achieve their highest capacity.

Appleton, a city of 50,000, has made a start in breaking the chronological lockstep in education. Its school administration has not been content with platitudes.

For years educators have hailed the doctrine of individual differences between children. It has been widely accepted that boys and girls progress at different rates of speed with bursts of achievement followed by interludes of apathy.

Dean Willard C. Olson of the University of Michigan has put it succinctly: ". . . individual differences in children are lawful expressions of designs for growing."

Though educators have paid lip service to this point of view they have continued to lump individuals together on the basis of age. The first-graders line up at the starting point at age six regardless of maturity or ability and march together year after year with little regard for their uniqueness as individuals. Ability grouping provides in some degree for these differences but grade levels are rigid structures which do not topple regardless of talent.

In many schools children who have completed curriculum requirements before the end of the year are not allowed to progress beyond their grade. This kind of progress complicates matters for next year's teacher, the school principal and the librarian. Life is simpler for the administrator when children move forward with chronological uniformity.

The "pass or fail" pressures of the September to June grade system have long seemed unhealthy to many educators. A slow-starter may receive an unwarranted brand as a failure and an A, B, C, D type of report card may reveal nothing of the individual's capabilities.

### Breaking With Tradition

Appleton's Continuous Progress Plan breaks with the traditions of September to June, "pass or fail" and uniformity. It is moving slowly toward eliminating age barriers but rapidly toward respect for individual differences. The homegrown plan, executed at no additional cost, is disarmingly simple.

After one year of kindergarten, children enter primary school for a three-year program. They are not given grade labels but are expected to complete an impressive academic program during the three-year bloc. Parents are informed about their children's strengths and weaknesses during a minimum of two parent-teacher conferences and by a midyear progress report. The progress report lists no numerical or alphabetical marks and contains no endless checklists of social and emotional characteristics. It describes with clarity the child's performance in relation to his capacity.

After completing three years of primary school, the Appleton youngster begins three years of intermediate school. A continuing battery of achievement tests enables the teacher to pinpoint the child's accomplishments and failings at parent-teacher conferences. During the final year of intermediate school the student participates in these conferences.

Most youngsters enter junior high school after this seven-year period but those who reveal immaturity or academic deficiencies may remain in either the primary or intermediate bloc for an extra year. Usually the decision to spend the extra year is made before the end of the term to lessen its impact on the child. Teachers discuss this with both the parents and the children.

Under Continuous Progress less than one half of 1 per cent of the students remain an additional year. Before the plan went into effect, Appleton's failure rate under the conventional graded system ranged from about 5 per cent in the 1922-35 period to about 2 per cent in 1951.

Does this mean that Appleton children are being coddled, that they are not being prepared for the realities of life?

According to standardized achievement tests they are outperforming their predecessors in graded classes and are exceeding national norms in all subjects.

In 1958 intermediate students made higher scores in the California Achievement Tests in reading, arithmetic and language arts than the Appleton youngsters of 1948. What's more, the level seems to be rising.

In 1956 children in their first year of intermediate school exceeded the national norm in total achievement by six months. In 1957 the same group increased its margin to seven months and in 1958, before entering junior high school, they were a full year and one month above the national median.

### Focus on the Individual

Appleton's respect for individual differences begins before a child reaches kindergarten age. Children whose fifth birthday occurs before September 1 enter kindergarten automatically, but special provision is made for advanced youngsters with September, October and November birthdays. Parents are notified that these underage children are eligible for testing to determine whether they are ready for school. The tests are not mandatory and some parents prefer to wait the extra year. In 1959, 227 youngsters were examined and 106 were accepted for early admission to kindergarten.

Follow-up studies of the young entrants of the past reveal their high performance. Twenty-nine of the 46 early admission students completing Appleton elementary schools in 1959 ranked in the first of four reading groups; 10 were in the second; 7 in the third; none in the fourth.

Appleton youngsters attend conventional-sized classes and their self-contained classrooms are of the familiar pattern. When schools have more than one class of the same level, students are grouped according to maturity. They may be shifted from one room to another during the year. Within each room they are divided again into small groups for reading, spelling and arithmetic. Each child has his individual skill card.

The skill card is a four-page folder on which the child's scholastic progress is charted. It breaks down arithmetic skills to be mastered during the six years of primary and intermediate school but there are no target dates listed. Entries are made by teachers when the skill is first introduced and later mastered. There are similar sections in reading and spelling. The skill card, a vivid picture of continuous progress, is passed from teacher to teacher until the youngster reaches junior high school. At the beginning of each new term the teacher simply picks up where her predecessor ended.

Appleton teachers and principals are discovering the same delightful truths that characterize experimentation all over the United States. When children and teachers are free to probe beyond limits established by administrative convenience, their potential soars.

There is a boy at the Foster School who read fluently while in kindergarten. When he began primary school his advanced reading status did not embarrass his teacher. She has assigned him responsibilities which put his talent to work without singling him out obtrusively. Periodically he reads a list of books lent to his class by the public library and collects them for return.

When he brought a caterpillar to class his teacher assigned him to find and read a book describing the development of butterflies and moths.

This boy is not held back because the rest of the class has not yet learned to read. On the other hand, he is not pushed ahead on all fronts.

He is immature in many ways [says his teacher], and he wants to remain with his group. His arithmetic concepts are not advanced and he's uncomfortable with older boys and girls. Six or seven other children are developing reading skills rapidly and eventually he'll have plenty of companionship. Meanwhile he's moving ahead with his reading without being segregated from his friends.

Asked about her reaction to Continuous Progress, she replied:

I think it's wonderful psychologically. I'm not conscious of June any more as the month that spells success or failure. We're concerned about progress during a three-year period, not about the ups and downs of a child's schooling during the next few months. The skill cards enable us to give new work to the advanced youngsters instead of "busy work" to fill the time until the slower children catch up.

## *Discovery Is the Keynote*

Youngsters who are ready for work beyond primary school level are encouraged to tackle intermediate subjects. A group of primary boys and girls at Huntley School who had read more than 30 books listed on their skill cards completed as many as 50 additional volumes in early 1959. This self-selection process, which is encouraged in all Appleton schools, is designed to stimulate self-direction and a sense of discovery. In November 1959 the group began reading intermediate material although they do not become intermediates officially until September 1960.

The same is true in arithmetic. Twelve Huntley youngsters, having completed primary work in November 1959 and ranking in the top 10 per cent of arithmetic students based on national test results, have launched intermediate work instead of delaying for the starting-gun in September of 1960. When they reach intermediate school their teachers will inherit advanced students with advanced skill cards and there will be no lost motion in discovering their talents.

Discovery is also a keynote of Appleton's parent-teacher conferences. There is nothing unusual about voluntary meetings but Appleton's insistence on a minimum of two conferences a year has proved highly effective. For one thing some parents come to school only when summoned. For another, problems come to light which might never have been recognized.

There was a boy in my class [a teacher reported recently] who seemed suddenly to be in a state of shock. He was silent, stared straight ahead, refused to participate in classroom discussions. There was no explanation from home but the boy's mother was due for a regular conference so I didn't contact her. When she came to see me I told her about ——'s sudden change.

"Didn't he tell you about his grandfather's death?" she asked. "—— was terribly close to his grandfather because his father travels a great deal and they did many things together while my husband was on the road. When his grandfather died the bottom just dropped out of his world."

If it weren't for that meeting with the mother [added the teacher], I might have pressured —— and it would have been just the wrong thing at that time. If a youngster's parent dies we usually hear of it at school and we're prepared to understand his reaction but other deaths in the family or more subtle matters rarely reach us except at conferences.

### Value of Conferences

Conferences enable teachers to present parents with a realistic picture of their youngsters' attainments at school.

"Profiles" of each child show his standing in reading vocabulary, reading comprehension, arithmetic reasoning, arithmetic fundamentals, mechanics of English and spelling in relation to national norms and the record of his own group. By comparing the child's mental capacity with his actual achievement, parent and teacher can see visually whether he is achieving his full capabilities.

The participation of students in the final conference of the intermediate school has proved a great success. It gives them a realistic look at their assets and liabilities as they are about to enter junior high school. Questionnaires were sent to 380 families requesting their reaction to the parent-teacher-child meetings; 272 replied.

*Question* 1

Did you like the idea of having your child participate in the final spring conference?

Yes—268; No—4

*Question* 2

Did your child express a willingness to participate in the conference?

Eager—113; Willing—138; Indifferent—11; Reluctant—7; Unwilling—6

*Question* 3

What was your child's reaction following the conference?

Pleased—163; Enthusiastic—23; Indifferent—9; More Informed—97

*Question* 4

Do you feel this three-way method of conferring has merit and should be continued as a means of developing mutual understanding?

Yes—265; No—7

*Note:*

Some parents checked more than one blank in questions 2 and 3.

Appleton teachers believe that conferences and progress reports provide more meaningful appraisal of a youngster than the naked marks on a report card.

In April 1959 a survey of unsigned teacher opinions revealed that of 73 primary and intermediate teachers who had taught in both A, B, C, and progress reporting systems, 69 *preferred* the progress report.

### *Progress Report Versus Report Cards*

Supporters of progress reporting point out that traditional report cards assume that all children are alike and are striving for the same goals. Adults, they say, never attempt to compare the work of a teacher, a mechanic and a physician, but adherents of numerical or alphabetical marking do not recognize the inborn differences of children.

Report cards purport to be based on a fixed standard but the standards vary from teacher to teacher. Even if the standard is fixed accurately, a "mark" can only compare a youngster to the rest of the group and may have no relation to his potential. The report card, its critics conclude, tends to bring undue pressure on the slower pupils while it fails to challenge the more gifted student.

The Appleton progress report form provides parents with a large space in which to write their comments. A recent examination of hundreds of these statements revealed that fewer than ten preferred a return to the conventional report card. The opinions of the overwhelming majority are reflected by these two comments:

You really know our ——! Both of us feel you've hit the nail on the head in most all of your statements. We feel —— is extremely fortunate to have a teacher who knows him well and understands how to cope with his boundless energy. . . .

We are deeply grateful for the intelligent, sensitive teaching that —— is receiving this year. Surely it reaches far beyond the mechanics of the teaching profession. We know that —— will long remember intermediate I as one of the happiest of all, for it has been a year free of pressure and tension yet one in which he appears to be making steady progress at a healthy rate of speed.

The Continuous Progress Plan is still at an early stage of its development. Its full potential has not been realized and Appleton school officials are the first to point this out. One of the richest possibilities lies in mixed grouping. This would bring together in the same room children of varied ages. Today the bright students forge ahead within the same classroom as less gifted youngsters of the same age. Appleton teachers point out that in many instances this is desirable because the student who is academically advanced may be immature socially and require the companionship of classmates of the same age.

They hasten to add, however, that the fulfillment of their belief that children can proceed at their own pace would be the elimination of arbitrary boundaries between the various years of primary and intermediate school. They accept the fact that many gifted children are mature enough to work with older classmates.

When Appleton solves this problem it will have broken the chronological lockstep completely. At the moment there are thirteen mixed group classes blending youngsters separated by at least one year of school experience.

At the Edison School a skilled teacher is experimenting with a class containing children of the first and second years of primary school. Preliminary results are excellent. She has found that the age span of more than two years has not hindered the rapid progress of small groups of pupils working with remarkable independence.

Appleton educators are coming to grips with other problems. Superintendent of Schools J. P. Mann points out that "the development of our Continuous Progress Plan will have a marked effect on the educational program in the junior and senior high schools."

Under Continuous Progress gifted intermediate students begin junior high school work before completing their sixth year of elementary school. This has influenced junior high schools to adjust their programs to avoid wasting time in repetition. Visitors to Appleton point out that if Continuous Progress is desirable for the elementary school, a comparable philosophy may be equally useful for junior and senior high school.

A healthy atmosphere for experimentation exists in Appleton and the next few years are likely to see exciting developments in its schools.

Superintendent Mann says that the driving force behind Continuous Progress has been the city's director of elementary education, Martha Sorensen. Her graduate work at Northwestern University concentrated on the individual differences of children, a subject to which she has devoted much of her educational career.

The facts are [says Miss Sorensen] that children differ in many ways. The school must accept, respect and provide for these differences. This simply means that educational machinery must be flexible, materials of instruction varied, the means for learning many and the practices in tune with what we know about how children grow and develop.

Miss Sorensen first stimulated the community's interest with a study of its failures under the graded system and in 1947 other teachers joined her in considering organizational and reporting plans that would be based on the differences rather than the similarities of children.

By 1951 parents and school board members, as well as teachers, were considering the new program. That September it was established on an experimental basis with first-year students in one school. The following year it was extended to the beginning primary students at all schools. In 1957-58 the program was adopted throughout the elementary schools. No additional costs have been involved.

In their valuable work *The Nongraded Elementary School* Professors John I. Goodlad and Robert H. Anderson describe The School We Could Have:

The facts and theory that suggest the kind of elementary school we advocate are largely a product of the twentieth century. The circumstances that led to the elementary school which we would abolish were characteristic of the nineteenth century. We believe that research on human development, learning, and curriculum, now available to educators, points to a nongraded type of elementary school organization.

Appleton appears to have made a good start.

## PROJECT HEAD START: AN ASSESSMENT [3]

PROJECT HEAD START:

  —is administered by the Office of Economic Opportunity as
    part of the War on Poverty.
  —is designed to break the cycle of poverty at its most critical
    point: during a child's formative years.
  —has so far touched the lives of 1.3 million disadvantaged
    children.
  —operates two kinds of programs: (1) eight-week-long sum-
    mer programs for four- and five-year-olds who will enter
    school the following fall; (2) a "full-year" program
    (lasting anywhere from three to twelve months) for
    three-, four-, and five-year-olds.
  —contains five major components: (1) health services, in-
    cluding medical exams, sight and hearing tests, dental
    exams, immunizations; (2) nutrition supplementation
    which includes one and often two full meals a day; (3)
    education, with emphasis placed on doing, rather than
    listening, in classes limited to fifteen children with one
    teacher and two teacher aides; (4) parent involvement as
    participants in all activities in the centers, on advisory
    councils, and as paid or volunteer nonprofessional staff
    members; (5) social services including interviews with
    parents, recommendation for family counseling services,
    or referral to public housing authorities, social hygiene
    departments, or church counseling services.

Head start is great [exults a Vermont Head Start teacher]. It gives
the kid freedom—a chance to run and jump and get hot. But if after a
summer of this he's suddenly thrown into a school system that allows no
kind of freedom, where he's told to sit down and shut up . . . well, it's
bound to confuse him and make him wonder what school is all about. I
think that maybe the biggest thing that can come from Head Start is that
our first and second grade education will be liberalized so that children will
have more individual freedom. We hope this will be a challenge to the
teachers. It certainly is a challenge to the conservative, classical, middle-
class concepts of what is right in education.

[3] From "Head Start or False Start?" by Charles S. Carleton, staff writer. *American Education*. 2:20-2. S. '66. *American Education* is a publication of the United States Office of Education.

These candid observations are not unique to the Green Mountain State. They are being echoed across the country as hundreds of thousands of Head Start youngsters pour into regular kindergarten and first-grade classrooms.

There is no doubt that Head Start is working, that for disadvantaged children it means entering regular school better prepared, with greater self-confidence and with a considerably advanced mental capacity compared to children from the same background without Head Start training. (In fact, Benjamin S. Bloom, professor of education at the University of Chicago, says that half of a seventeen-year-old's mental ability is developed by the time he is four years old—just the age group that Head Start brackets.)

Perhaps the most significant boost that Head Start children are given is their introduction to the world of words. Coming from homes without books, where English is spoken poorly if at all, this vocabulary expansion (both in terms of exposure and actual use) gives them a real jump in their ability to learn through reading and conversation.

But unless Head Start is followed through in the classroom it can be meaningless; or worse, it can be a false start. How?

Well, as one Head Start teacher puts it:

It's not that the regular teachers push them back down but, unless the teachers are better than average, they do cut off the gay, inquiring spirit that these kids have been taught. In fact, there were teachers last year who complained they had to have the Head Start kids be quiet while they brought the rest of the children up to their level.

Although having Head Starters get such a jump that they are ahead of their more fortunate peers is unique—and common sense dictates against an eight-week summer program's making up for four or five years of lost ground—Head Starters are set apart in many ways from their peers. A Head Start child's health problems have been taken care of; he is accustomed to receiving breakfast and/or lunch as part of the school day; he is used to a good deal of personal attention when he needs help, and, as a result, he probably is more easily distracted and less persistent in his activities than other children—more inclined to nonconformism—all traits that indicate a heightening of self-esteem, a growing curiosity, and increasing intellectual development. Additionally, the Head Start child receives more support for his school activities at home than his classmates because of the direct, personal contact with parents that Head Start encourages. As a result of this contact parents are likely to feel that the schools are interested in them and in what they have to say. In exchange, they are more willing to put out some effort on behalf of the schools.

Comments the Vermont teacher:

Of course, the kids have to adjust when they switch from Head Start to school because in a lot of cases they're taking a step backwards. But it's not going to ruin them. Our first grade teachers are slowly coming to appreciate what Head Start is doing. And the kids who can't adjust to the change are the ones who aren't capable of adjusting to anything anyway. But most of them can adjust—because kids are smart; they know which way the wind blows. Anyway, we have to make the effort. You know what Eleanor Roosevelt said: "It's better to light a candle than to curse the darkness."

## *Importance of Follow-up*

To keep the Head Start candle burning, school systems and Head Start personnel need to work together, exchanging ideas and information, and searching for possible areas of accommodation.

Teachers and administrators should know what is happening in their community Head Start program so they will have a better idea of what kind of children they will be taking into their schools come September. Head Start centers generally welcome visitors to their classes—and certainly should, since the child gains so much from the visit.

Conversely, Head Start personnel should learn just what experiences their children will be having when they go on to school so they can operate the program within a realistic framework. This is not to say that Head Start should be an earlier version of school. In fact, many experts discourage the notion of prepping a child for kindergarten or first grade activities, suggesting that it is not as important for the child to learn to cut, paste, and color as for him to be made comfortable with and attracted to the notion that he can create. Similarly, he should get a feeling for music, rather than learn a specific number of songs. In short, Head Start should take positive steps to move the child into school with a healthy, excited attitude about the new experience—and with an awareness of how it will be different from Head Start.

Additionally, the school system should do some soul searching for ways it can improve itself.

What is being done to individualize instruction for each child? The promising ungraded primary system is slowly gaining popularity. Other techniques include expanded use of team teaching, teaching machines, and programed instruction.

Are changes in teaching style in order? For example, is a greater variety of materials and resources needed? Can a greater number of activities be carried on simultaneously in the classroom?

Is there a large enough staff working with the younger children? Here the use of Title I, ESEA [Elementary and Secondary Education Act—see Section III, above] funds may offer opportunities for reducing class size or employing nonprofessional teacher aides. Further help may be available by making greater use of volunteers.

How can the interest of parents be maintained and expanded? Can the operation of the PTA be changed to create a more helpful dialogue between the schools and parents? How can the health and nutritional gains of the child be maintained? Other Federal funds such as those available through the Children's Bureau, Special Project Grants, and the Social Security Act, may be useful in providing continuous health care.

In what ways might the school's and teacher's roles change in working with the the total family? To what extent can a school assume social service responsibilities?

How can we assure that all disadvantaged children's cultural horizons will continue to expand?

Perhaps most important and fundamental to all program changes is the matter of teacher acceptance of Head Start. One school system's teachers were dead set against Head Start because they feared that the children would come to class like a horde of miniature Huns, destroying everything in sight because they lacked discipline. As it turned out, these worst fears were not realized; on the contrary, the children, because of their Head Start experience, were ready to take instructions and work placidly with one another.

More important than the attitude the teacher may have about the Head Start program is the teacher's attitude toward the child. Schools and teachers should ask themselves if they are doing their utmost to see the unique opportunities to help the child and increase his optimism for the future. Children feel deeply the expectations of their teachers. If the teacher believes the child is already lost, he probably will be; if the teacher believes he has a bright future, he probably will.

One of the most important—and time consuming—lessons that can be learned from Head Start is how much good can come from the involvement of teachers with parents in an effort to help the child. Says one teacher:

I had a boy in my class who was a real problem. He pushed the other children around, actually attacked them, and just gave me a very rough time. Then I found out that his father beats his mother, and the child lives in mortal terror of it. There are six children in the family, and the father feels trapped and takes it out on beer, babes, and beating momma. Well, I've talked with them and I've worked with the child. But the usual kindergarten teacher can't give a child like that the kind of individual attention he needs. She's by herself and she's got thirty other children to take care of. Head Start made it possible for this boy to come and have a sort of play therapy for four hours a day. I think he'll hang on to some of it. Luckily he's going in with a teacher who understands this kind of problem and may be able to help him.

## Avoiding Pitfalls

In Baltimore's large (1,140 children this past summer) Head Start program, many of the possible pitfalls have been avoided through sound organization and accurate foresight. Mrs. Elaine Nolan, director of the program, says that before they got started they were aware that there could be some adjustment problems for the children when they went on to school. So, all of her Head Start teachers are regular teachers taken from the school system's kindergarten classes. "That way," she explains, "we can have the teacher who has worked with the children during the summer teach the class in September."

The Baltimore schools also make use of teacher aides and volunteers so that more individual instruction is possible.

And [says Mrs. Nolan], we found that by grouping the Head Start children together, the child's adjustment to the school situation has been helped rather than hindered by the summer program. We didn't use teacher aides in the school before Head Start. Our teachers felt they had much more success in this program than in any other they had been a part of. The services available to the children over the summer gave them the advantage of knowing problems in advance.

All over the nation, Head Start is having its impact—is lighting, and keeping lit, those candles. Approximately 20 per cent of the nation—some 35 million people—live under adverse circumstances. Of these, 17 million are children. As a consequence of Head Start, communities all over America are now vitally concerned with the problems of the children of "not-enough." We have developed a national awareness that they can be helped, and that this is the time to do it.

During last year's summer program nearly half of the more than three thousand counties in the nation had at least one Head Start center, thereby taking the first vital step in breaking the cycle of poverty, laying a foundation for a lifetime of learning, for better jobs, and often for better health.

The results?

I see more children less tearful, less fearful [writes a Head Start teacher]. I see more smiles, more working together wtih classmates and adults. I see more verbal expression. The interaction of the child with a helpful adult may be the most important factor in all these gains.

It is important to realize that these first steps taken by Head Start should not be final steps [says Minnie Berson, Office of Education specialist in early childhood education]. With cooperation and planning, with dedication and understanding, with a willingness to extend the gains of Head Start, our schools can help—and continue to help—every child of poverty. The child whose future is made brighter by Head Start need not have that light extinguished.

## ONE CAMPUS FOR ALL SCHOOLS? [4]

A new approach to education, little noticed outside professional circles, is beginning to spread across the country. In city after city, groups of elementary and high schools are being built together on downtown campuses, much like those of colleges.

These campuses are given such names as "educational parks" or "school villages." They are largely the result of a nationwide search for better means of public education.

Some are all at the high school level; others range from kindergarten through junior college. Enrollment runs into the thousands. Usually the students are divided into a number of smaller units, called "houses," or "halls." School spirit focuses on the house or hall.

One principal purpose is to provide, for the consolidated smaller schools, the advantages of a big school—the special teachers, wider range of courses, and the modern mechanical and electronic equipment which the small school usually cannot afford.

Another objective, in some cities, is to combat "downtown blight." By establishing attractive schools of high quality in downtown areas, cities hope to encourage families to halt or reverse the flight to the suburbs.

In other cities, a primary aim is to end so-called de facto segregation. Pupils in large schools are drawn from a wider area. Pockets of school segregation caused by the predominance of Negroes or whites in one neighborhood are wiped out.

The larger school has suddenly come into favor [says Dr. Harold B. Gores, president of the Educational Facilities Laboratories, an organization established by the Ford Foundation for educational research]. Until recently, the accepted theory was that schools should have no more than seven hundred to twelve hundred students, to avoid "the sense of anonymity and facelessness."

As our nation doubles in population, schools will necessarily be larger than in the old days we have known. Indeed, the consolidation of schools is going on all over the country, providing greater efficiency, more and better service by virtue of their centralization.

[4] From "One Campus for All Schools—Is This Your City's Solution?" *U.S. News & World Report.* 58:53-6. Je. 14, '65. Reprinted from *U.S. News & World Report,* published at Washington.

## Economical Concentration

This is what is happening:

In northwestern New York State, at Youngstown, an elaborate educational park has been in existence for more than ten years. The school district purchased three farms, totaling 365 acres, and built all of its elementary and high schools on the land, with the exception of classrooms for kindergarten through third grade. Three thousand students now attend school in the group of three buildings on the campus.

The school district has found this concentration economical, and at the same time the quality of education has been improved. Expensive facilities can be used jointly. Better teachers have been attracted to the improved schools.

For the past two years, a similar complex has been in operation in Golden Valley, a suburb of Minneapolis. On a 47.5-acre tract with a lake and stream are schools for the district's 1,500 pupils in grades five through high school.

In Evanston, Illinois, a high school campus for a student body of 6,000 is being developed. The high school now has 4,329 students. Five buildings are to house the institution, on a 53-acre site.

Students are enrolled in "halls," called North, South, East and West.

Each hall has its own principal and operates semi-independently. Evanston bunched its high school program into the one site to use the tract of land available and because of the advantages of a big-school operation.

Near Fort Lauderdale, Florida, Broward County is developing what it calls the South Florida Educational Center. On a 320-acre site, formerly a military airport, the county has built a high school and junior college. An elementary school, now under construction, will open in September. Later, a university is to be added.

The purpose of this complex is described as an effort to develop better educational methods. It will be a kind of demonstration school and educational laboratory.

A similar experimental complex has been established in Bloomington, Indiana, as a joint project of the city and Indiana University.

Called the University Schools, it has 13 buildings on a 43-acre campus, with pupils ranging from preschool through high school.

Southfield, Michigan, a suburb of Detroit, has gathered all of its senior high school students, grades 10 through 12, on a 70-acre campus. It now has 2,200 students, will have 3,000 when fully developed. Two classroom buildings and a library are on the site, and a third classroom building is under construction. All are connected by glass-enclosed corridors.

Students are enrolled in three "houses." Each house has its own supervisor and three counselors, and its own cafeteria. All are under one principal.

"We have tried to capture the advantage of the smaller school in a larger context," says Dr. John English, superintendent of schools at Southfield. The school has a complete vocational education program, including electronics and drafting classes, plus a number of advanced science courses.

### Big-School Variety

Boston is planning a campus high school for 5,500 students. It is to be on a 35-acre site in the central part of the city, probably in an urban-renewal area. One of the motives is to help rehabilitate downtown Boston by establishing a school of unusually high standards.

It will offer a wide range of technical, vocational and academic subjects which are intended to attract students from throughout the city. The curriculum will provide courses and activities that a small school could not offer, such as lessons in the performing arts. Its name will be the Central Boston Secondary Education Complex.

Boston also is considering educational parks for its elementary schools, some of which have been criticized for their de facto segregation.

The practice of dividing large high schools into smaller student bodies was begun in 1959 at Newton, Massachusetts. With 4,000 high school students in groups of buildings on two separate campuses, it has split up the students into nine "houses." Each house is named for some well-known educator.

East Orange, New Jersey, is planning to convert its entire school system into one downtown "educational plaza." On a 15-acre site next to a 12-acre park, it will put up eight buildings for 10,000 students, from kindergarten through junior college. Its present thirteen schools will be sold to help pay for the plaza.

First step will be construction of one building, for 3,000 pupils in grades 5 through 8. Ground for this school will be broken in the spring of 1966. Later construction will take place over a twelve-to-fifteen-year period at a cost of about $35 million. The new school plaza will be a community center, open the year round, day and night. It will provide adult classes, recreation and facilities for community activities.

It will be possible for most students to walk to the plaza, since it is within 1.5 miles of most homes in East Orange. Motives of the school planners are typical—getting new school buildings, curing downtown blight and eliminating pockets of de facto segregation. Sixty per cent of public-school students in East Orange are Negroes.

## TV, Special Classes

On a 140-acre tract in Sarasota, Florida, the first element of an educational park, called the McIntosh Student Center, has been built. Eventually, all of Sarasota's schools will be situated there. Three more buildings are to be added, covering first grade through junior college.

The Sarasota center will offer many new devices, including closed-circuit television, language laboratories, remedial teaching and special classes for gifted students.

The Pittsburgh board of education has given general approval for three or four educational-park complexes, probably the largest such project being planned. Each will have schools for 10,000 to 25,000 students. Each will consist of a central park, surrounded by satellite parks—within walking distance of each other and connected by "greenways."

At the core will be a junior college and high school. Farther out will be the "middle schools," grades 6 through 8. In parks still farther removed from the central section will be the lower elementary schools. Altogether, there will be eight or ten buildings in each complex of parks. In addition, on the periphery will be a series of prekindergarten schools, perhaps in restored homes.

Pittsburgh's plan is to raze or rehabilitate blighted areas on a large scale. Between the educational parks, and between the schools within each park, new housing developments will be built.

"The schools will be the focal points for new neighborhoods," says Dr. Sidney Marland, superintendent of Pittsburgh schools. "These will be distinguished schools. Families will want to live near them so as to take advantage of the superior education they will offer."

New York City school officials also are studying a proposal to create three educational parks for a number of its "middle schools," grades 5 through 8. The aim there would be to overcome de facto segregation as well as to provide better educational facilities.

The New York plan would put about 15,000 pupils in each park, then subdivide these into schools of 500 to 1,000 pupils each.

Sites for the parks in the Bronx and Brooklyn are under consideration.

Some educators see educational parks as helpful in developing "shared time" programs. In these, parochial school students are released from their own schools to attend certain classes in public schools, thus relieving the parochial schools of part of the rising costs of education.

Each community has its own reasons for refashioning its public schools. But more and more of them are finding that big downtown schools, or school parks, villages or plazas are the answer to local problems.

## MAKING SUMMER SCHOOL COUNT [5]

It was a warm summer day and the murmur of rustling leaves outside mingled with the murmur of voices in the classroom.

[5] From "From Maine to California: Revolution in Summer Schools," by Benjamin H. Pearse, a staff writer in the United States Office of Education's Office of Information. *American Education*. 2:10-12. O. '66. *American Education* is a publication of the United States Office of Education.

"The pen red—" the boy began, translating from his French reader.

The teacher shook his head. "In English, Marcel, it is 'the red pen'; remember?"

Marcel nodded sheepishly and started over. "The red pen is on the *tahbl.*"

"That's better, but in English we say *taybul,* not *tahbl.* Try again."

Marcel repeated the sentence, correctly this time, and sat down amid the approving giggles of some twenty youngsters who repeated the words softly until the teacher called on the next pupil.

This classroom full of children learning English is not in Paris or Quebec, nor are the children French or Canadian. All are American, born and raised in Escourt Station on the Maine side of the Canadian border, trying to learn their "native" tongue, English. But let their teacher, Peter Toschi, explain.

The American community in Escourt Station is smaller than the Canadian town of Escourt, New Brunswick, and so the American youngsters have been attending school on the Canadian side. The instruction there is in French, of course, except for one hour a day of English to meet the requirements of the bilingual school system. The result is a patois more French than English.

The summer school started five years ago at the request of parents, Americans of French extraction, who did not speak English very well themselves and wanted their children to know their official language. The Maine State Department of Education rented a hall in back of the post office building and hired Mr. Toschi, a school principal during the regular term, to teach the six-week summer session. This year it also furnished textbooks.

When I call the roll [Mr. Toschi told me], I'm not sure which side of the border I'm on. There are three Gagne girls, six of the Sirois family, six Theriault children, four Desjardins, and the Levesque youngster. But they're gradually losing their French idiom. They talk more like Americans every day.

### Boom in Summer Schooling

Summer schools have been a regular feature at colleges and universities for decades but summer sessions at grade and high schools are a relatively recent development. A survey of elementary education a decade ago ignored elementary summer sessions altogether because there were so few of them. When the elementary summer school movement began to gain momentum five or six years ago, courses were largely remedial, offering students who flunked a regular school subject a chance to catch up before fall. The extra sessions have become so popular, however, that advanced courses have been added, as well as subjects not included in the regular term.

On the basis of a nationwide survey conducted by the National Education Association, it is estimated that eighteen thousand public high schools conducted summer sessions in 1966 with a total enrollment of about three million. No census of elementary school summer sessions has been made, but estimates are that attendance may have reached another million.

The NEA survey revealed a significant change in summer session curriculums. Although the great majority of subjects offered a decade ago were remedial and 67 per cent of today's schools still offer remedial courses, only 3 per cent offer only remedial courses. The others have added advanced courses in science and the humanities, in art and music. Some subjects are accepted for college credit.

Within the past few years, then, the character of summer sessions in grade and high schools has almost completely changed. The special sessions still offer a second chance for the slow learner or unmotivated student, but the main thrust is toward expanding the student's horizon, enriching his educational experience, and stimulating his intellectual appetite. This is no more than might be expected, perhaps, in the more affluent suburbs such as Beverly Hills, California, where 70 per cent of the students attend summer sessions, in Cleveland's Shaker Heights, or in communities on Long Island or Westchester County in New York. But now, with funds available under the Elementary and Secondary Education Act of 1965 (ESEA), it is also becoming characteristic of the low-income school districts throughout the nation where the need for stimulation and enrichment is much more pressing. Many school districts are learning that summer sessions offer an unusual opportunity, because of the relatively short sessions (six or eight weeks), to experiment with new methods, and to give greater attention to individual pupils by cutting class sizes. The summer project at Fayetteville, Arkansas School District No. 1 is a good example.

## A Pilot Project

With the help of an ESEA grant, the Fayetteville district established a supplementary education center in an outgrown junior high school building. This summer the center conducted a pilot project for 132 children. Students in the pilot project were underachievers from the seventh to ninth grades (in the twelve to seventeen age group). They lived in the four counties around Fayetteville and were brought in and returned home daily by bus.

We wanted to give them as much individual attention as possible [Miss Florence McCormick, director of the center, said], so we had twenty-four teachers, six counselors, a psychologist, and specialists in science, math, shop, art, music and dancing, two reading specialists, a librarian, a nurse, two home coordinators, and two adult advisers.

Parents were very important to our program. The coordinators were in constant contact with the home and the adult advisers handled the discussions and instruction (usually films on child problems) when the parents came to "class" at the center two nights a week. We felt that the parental interest would go a long way in encouraging the child.

The relatively large faculty, with one teacher for every three or four students, insured individual instruction in the academic subjects and also allowed time for interviews by counselors and the psychologist to root out the underlying cause for each youngster's lack of progress. Individual programs were balanced by two projects in which all the students participated.

The first group project was a Gilbert and Phillips musical, *Creatures of Impulse*. Students who did not win a part or qualify for the chorus helped build and paint scenery, or assisted in making costumes. The final performance won enthusiastic acclaim from the largely family audience.

The other group project greatly stimulated the youngsters' imaginations. It was a three-day trip to the state capital at Little Rock and to Tulsa, Oklahoma.

None of the children had seen a wide screen movie before, or eaten in a cafeteria with its dazzling choice of foods—they were especially taken by the array of desserts—or had ever stayed in a hotel. The trip was the favorite topic of conversation among the students for the rest of the session.

We won't be able to evaluate this pilot program [Miss McCormick said] until we see whether these students do better in the regular term this fall. But in the reading tests we gave at the beginning and the close of the summer session, there was a significant improvement, an average increase of better than five per cent.

I am sure we can count on the cooperation of the parents in the future. They were quite regular in their attendance at the evening meetings and seemed impressed with their responsibility in offering the children encouragement.

The whole faculty believes we are on the right track and that the program will give a real impetus to education throughout the district.

The project is being extended to other Fayetteville schools this fall and to other schools throughout the twelve county district as fast as teachers can be trained.

## For Children and Parents

Parents also figured importantly in a project conducted in the heart of Baltimore's inner city this past summer where 100 per cent of the residents are Negro. In this program, 570 children from grades 3, 4, and 5 attended an elementary school while 125 of their parents attended classes in a junior high school building next door.

"Our purpose in this dual arrangement," said Mrs. Leana Farrell, head teacher at the elementary school, "was to bring the parents into the school circle, to get them interested in education and show them its importance."

The elementary pupils were given a basic diet of reading and arithmetic heavily spiced with bus trips to parks, to points of historical interest, to a newspaper, and to a restaurant. A theater group presented a play in a "showmobile" on the school grounds, and the Baltimore Symphony Orchestra came down to rehearse. Activities were geared to the theme A World of Lively Living.

The school for parents involved considerable advance planning and solicitation by Lloyd McDonald, guidance chief at the junior high, and his staff. Most participants were mothers since the husbands were at work but eleven fathers working night shifts attended, including one who wanted to learn to sign his name, instead of an "X," to his boy's report card.

To free the parents to attend school, babysitters were arranged for some homes and a nursery was set up for children too young for the elementary school. Hot lunches were served.

Classwork for the parents consisted of an hour of reading, half an hour of arithmetic, and an hour of discussion on municipal problems of special interest to them—rodent control, garbage collection, voter registration, police responsibilities. Representatives of the city government and civic organizations furnished lively leadership. Special classes were held for thirty-eight parents who could neither read nor write; many of them learned to do both in the six-week session. With the staff of eight teachers and eight discussion leaders, classes were held to a maximum of ten.

## Salvaging Dropouts

In Orange County, California, a joint campaign to salvage dropouts reported outstanding success last summer. While most of the county's school districts conducted sessions as usual, they also operated a junior and senior high school in Anaheim and a senior high school in Costa Mesa as a special dropout program. By dint of considerable canvassing of recent "withdrawal" rosters, enrollment reached close to one hundred at each of the three schools, and attendance during the eight-week term ranged from eighty-five to ninety. Many students were from minority groups, mostly Negroes and youngsters of Latin American and Japanese descent. More than a score of students registered without personal solicitation, after hearing about the school from friends or reading about it in newspapers.

One of the striking things [said Mrs. Naoma Troxell, supervisor of health and guidance] was the health inventory, which showed that 45 per cent of the students had pressing medical needs, some of them critical. It helped to explain many of the dropouts. But in general, most of our youngsters had acquired the motivation they lacked when they dropped out.

For example, a nineteen-year-old girl made her way on crutches to enroll. She had quit school in the eighth grade and most of the time since had been working in the fields as a farm laborer. She gave up her job to reenter high school this fall.

One of the most unusual summer schools was conducted on the Alamo Navajo Reservation about thirty-five miles from Magdalena, New Mexico. During the regular term, children from the Alamo reservation attended the Magdalena schools, staying at a dormitory provided by the Bureau of Indian Affairs.

The young children entering the first grade usually can't speak a word of English, Superintendent J. Buck Doran explained. It takes time for them to catch up, since during summer vacation they normally go back to the reservation where they hear and speak nothing but Navajo. Up to last year (1965), only two boys and three girls had graduated from Magdalena High School.

Our summer school was intended to keep the Alamo children in touch with books, and reading, and especially English [Superintendent Doran said]. It's very easy to forget a foreign language when you don't use it, and to the young Indians English is a foreign language.

Two trailers were purchased with ESEA funds, one for a classroom, the other furnished as living quarters for the teacher, Miss Florence Brown. The trailers were parked for two-week periods at each of five Indian encampments during the summer months.

My classroom could hold about twenty elementary children [Miss Brown said], and it was filled every morning. The ten or twelve secondary students were also quite regular in attendance and usually when class was over (about 4:30 in the afternoon) some of the boys who had been herding sheep all day would come in to borrow books. Education is winning friends among the parents since the youngsters are getting far enough along to translate Department of Agriculture bulletins for them and help them fill out Government forms. Most of the youngsters are fond of music, and enjoy rock 'n' roll.

### Innovations on the Rise

All sorts of innovations were tried in summer schools in various parts of the country to meet new problems or cope with old ones. In upper New York State, four schools in Oswego County that did not have enough students to hold summer sessions of their own combined to hold a joint session at the Mexico Academy and Central School in Mexico, New York. The combined registration of about 350 made possible a broad curriculum including such staples as science and English and a dozen other subjects ranging from auto repair to music appreciation. In the Peninsula School District near Olympia, Washington, the curriculum included a twenty-day tour of the state's historic sites and attendance at a Shakespeare festival.

But the summer session at Escourt Station can claim a special distinction. In the final week of the session, parents of the attending youngsters held a meeting to which they invited Mr. Toschi and James L. Brown, state supervisor of elementary education. There they voted to organize a school district so they could get a year-round public school. Mr. Brown will ask the state legislature for a two-room school at a cost of $55,000.

It will certainly be the only school that grew out of a summer session, instead of vice versa.

## V. THE REVOLUTION IN METHODS

### EDITOR'S INTRODUCTION

The Dean of Harvard's Graduate School of Education has summed it up this way: "We have been dealt a new set of cards, and we must learn how to play with them." The new set includes new approaches to the learning process and new techniques for employing them. For almost a decade after the end of World War II, educators were kept busy simply trying to handle quantitative problems—the flood of new youngsters clamoring at the schoolhouse door and the rapid expansion of facilities and personnel systems to accommodate them. Only in the last few years have qualitative problems come to the fore and the voices of such reformers as James B. Conant, Jerome Bruner, Francis Keppel, John W. Gardner and Lawrence Cremin been heard in the land.

Today the concept of intelligence as a "fixed" or "given" quality in each child is being swept away by the revolution in teaching methods. Reformers are preaching that intelligence is a quality which in itself can be learned, and through the growing adoption of new methods of instruction they are trying to prove their point. "Discovery" learning is the key phrase. What with the modern "explosion of knowledge," it is no longer feasible simply to cram as many facts and figures as possible into young heads over a twelve-year period. The student must be given the means of "discovering" or finding answers for himself, the stress must shift from the *content* of knowledge to its *structure*. Such is the essence of the "new math," which seeks to advise the student on the structure of mathematics—its "whys"—instead of concentrating on a dreary list of rules to be memorized. Such an approach, argue the reformers, is inherently more exciting and interesting to the student himself.

This section is designed to give the reader a general introduction to the revolution in methods that is sweeping our elementary and secondary schools. The first article discusses new approaches to the teaching of English. The problems of "discovery" learning in this field are somewhat more complicated and of a different order from those in fields such as mathematics and physical science. The second article is a progress report on the "new math"—on the whole, an optimistic one. In the final article a writer for *Fortune* magazine summarizes the nature of the revolution going forward in American education today, focusing in particular on its technological phase.

## THE COMING REVOLUTION IN TEACHING ENGLISH [1]

Modern parents complain that they can't help the kids with their homework anymore. The senile gaffers of forty or fifty have been left far behind by the physical sciences with their arcane particles and space gibberish. The youngsters don't even do long division the way we did it in the 1920's and 1930's. For those thus bewildered, it is comforting to return to good old English grammar. In a world where the tables of multiplication shift treacherously underfoot, we touch solid bedrock in the eternal truth that a noun is the name of a person, place, or thing.

And it is true the grammar still taught in most American schools would look perfectly familiar to Bishop Robert Lowth, who published *A Short Introduction to English Grammar* in 1762. Nevertheless, traditional, or Latinical, or Lowthian grammar is under heavy fire from the new grammarians. There are almost as many sects among these innovators as there are in Christendom. But all of them have in common the desire to analyze language with the same rigorous precision with which the chemist analyzes compounds, and all are more or less mathematical in style. Some of their formulations look rather terrifying to the non-initiate.

[1] Article by Andrew Schiller, associate professor of English at the University of Illinois in Chicago. *Harper's Magazine.* 229:82-92. O. '64. Copyright © 1964 by Harper's Magazine, Inc. Reprinted from the October, 1964 issue of *Harper's Magazine* by permission of the author.

Here is one example:

Description: NP W + Af as A X as (NPV$_c$) NP Y # Z

$$\underbrace{\phantom{NP W}}_{1} \underbrace{\phantom{+ Af}}_{2} \quad \underbrace{\phantom{as A X as (NPV_c)}}_{3} \quad \underset{4}{\phantom{NP}} \quad \underset{5}{\phantom{Y # Z}}$$

Condition: $2 = 4 + 5$

If 3 includes NPV$_c$, 4 is not null

Change: $1 + 2 + 3 + 4 + 5 \rightarrow 1 + 2 + 3 + 4$

And now for another:

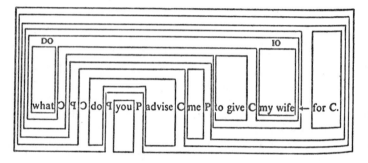

These formulations typify the two leading (and often contending) "schools" of modern linguistic thought. The first is known as transformational grammar. Its essential assumption is that language consists of irreducible kernel utterances, plus transformation laws, plus lexicon. The illustration is an abstract formula for generating sentences of the type, "John is taller than Bill."

The second example is from phrase-structure grammar (which some of the more condescending transformationalists are already calling "classical linguistics"). The interconnected boxes are a graphic device to show how the sentence, "What do you advise me to give my wife for Christmas?" is analyzed. To do this, you peel the grammatical construction apart by orderly stages, much as a mechanic disassembles an automobile into body, engine, cooling system, exhaust system, and running gear, these in turn into sub-assemblies, and so on to the ultimate constituents.

Taken undiluted, such grammars are sophisticated and difficult, strong drink for graduate students, not milk for children in the grades. But we do not teach school or college students linguistics; we teach them structural grammar which is based on what we have learned from linguistics. And I can report that youngsters who have been taught structural grammar (diluted, of course), have not only grasped but enjoyed it—an accomplishment comparable to making castor oil palatable. Generally, they are impressed by the ease with which a few principles cover a vast territory.

## The New Science of Language

Formulae of the kind shown above may seem far removed from the primary grades. But so are the equations of Einstein and Bohr. Yet modern grade schoolers prattle easily of orbits and weightlessness, atomic energy and space-time. In a like fashion, the concepts of modern linguistics, on which the new grammars are based, will one day filter down in a general, accessible form to most adults and children. So far this has not happened. But that is an accident of history. Structural linguistics—the exact science of language—is about three or four decades behind the physical sciences in this respect.

Around 1925, for example, physicists were already familiar with the theoretical basis of nuclear fission. No one could then have predicted that in twenty years the equations would be translated into a bomb, ten years later into a power plant—and that the average teen-ager of the 1950's and 1960's would be as glib with his physics as his parents had been with Freudian psychology. In the same fashion the new science of language is bound to erupt into the public consciousness. When that happens, much grammatical theory that has been passed from generation to generation in our schools, virtually unchanged for centuries, will be laid quietly in our intellectual attic alongside astrology and alchemy.

What—if any—will be the practical benefits? Will this new information from the linguists help us in our job of teaching reading and writing? I have no doubt that it will.

At present, the teacher of traditional grammar is at a serious disadvantage compared with the science teacher. In a chemistry class, for example, students learn that the electrolysis of water produces hydrogen and oxygen in the proportion of two to one. In the laboratory they verify this for themselves. But when the grammarian asserts that a sentence must consist of a subject and a predicate, and state a complete thought, his students cannot prove this for themselves. To begin with, we cannot precisely define a "complete thought." Take the sentence, "I am going to the concert." According to the grammarians, that is a complete thought. If "complete" has its ordinary meaning, then if we subtract something, what remains should be less than complete. But the statement, "I am going," is, according to the same grammarians, still a complete thought. So is "I am."

Nor does any particular form or shape or length of sentence distinguish a complete thought from an incomplete one.

The other classic criterion of a sentence is that it names a subject and predicates something about it. This is just as slippery. Consider the sentence, "The door is open." Here we have a subject and a predicate—a complete sentence. On the other hand, consider the phrase, "the open door." Have we not given the name of a thing, place, or person? Have we not stated something about that thing? Certainly the student cannot verify this definition for himself.

Now let us take a different approach. I say to someone, "The door is open." He may reply, "I'll close it." However, if I say, "The open door . . ." he simply waits for me to continue. If I fail to go on he will laugh, believing I have fallen asleep with my mouth open. He knew after the first utterance that I was finished, that some reply or action was expected of him. He knew after the second that I was not. This was not because I said less, but because the two utterances had different formal characteristics. Take another example. If I say to you, "This is the best," you know that you can now agree or disagree. But if I say, "This is the best . . ." you will not respond until I add best *what*.

These two utterances were word for word the same but you received two different sets of signals. The difference is not merely a matter of completion; in the second utterance you not only knew something else was coming, you knew exactly what sort of thing— namely a noun or some nominal expansion. That is, I could not possibly have completed the utterance with the word "very," but I could have completed it with "piano" or "of all possible worlds." From such examples the linguist concludes that it is not particularly useful to define a noun in terms of meaning. It is more useful to identify a class of words that can be placed at the end of the utterance, "This is the best . . ." He concludes also that the difference between a sentence and a non-sentence must be stated in terms other than meaning.

### Stress, Pitch, Juncture

What other criteria are there? Further analysis reveals three phenomena which together differentiate "This is the . . ." from "This is the best." These phenomena are stress, pitch, and juncture. Understanding how they function gives us an insight into the structural linguists' approach to language.

As to stress, in English speech four distinct degrees can readily be heard in such a phrase as "portable typewriter." The first syllable of each word is marked by a heavy stress, but—and this is the important distinction—not equally heavy. If you ask how I wrote this article, I reply, "I used a portable TYPEwriter." If on the other hand you ask what kind of typewriter I generally use, I say, "I use a PORTable typewriter." So we distinguish primary and secondary stress, marked respectively ´ and ^. Now if we listen to the word *typewriter* we can hear that the stress on the second syllable is lighter than the first but heavier than the third. This gives us the third and fourth degrees (tertiary and minimal) marked respectively ` and ˘ (though in actual transcriptions, minimals are usually left unmarked for simplicity). The two different stress patterns are indicated thus:

Q: How did you write this article?
A: I used a pôrtăblĕ týpewrìtĕr.

Q: What kind of typewriter do you generally use?
A: I use a pórtăblĕ tŷpewrìtĕr.

Note that the shift in stress is not random. Changes in stress affect meaning.

There are also four levels of pitch in English. Our first sentence would look like this on a musical staff:

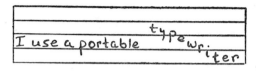

To replace the cumbersome staff, linguists express the pitch pattern in this grammatical notation:

$$2 \qquad\qquad 3 \qquad 1$$
I use a portable typewriter.

Suppose now that I am not going to finish the sentence with the word "typewriter"—perhaps I will continue with the clause, "since I work while I travel." You now hear:

$$2 \qquad\qquad 3 \qquad 2$$
I use a portable typewriter

and you know that I am not finished. If I were dictating, you would use a comma after the word "typewriter." On the other hand, suppose I said:

$$2 \qquad\qquad 3 \qquad 3$$
I use a portable typewriter

the so-called rising inflection would tell you that I was finished and had asked a question.

Pitch four is commonly used *in extremis* to indicate intense emphasis, alarm, indignation, such as:

$$2 \qquad\qquad 4 \qquad 1$$
Come here this instant!

A stream of speech is composed not only of sounds but of breaks in the succession of sounds. These gaps are of specific types and come in specific places. They are part of the grammar of the utterance, like nouns and verbs, and this pitch-pause phenomenon is known as juncture.

One type of juncture enables us to distinguish "announce" from "an ounce." In "announce" the sounds are all hooked together without a break. But in "an ounce" there is a break between the second and third sounds. The same phenomenon occurs in such pairs as "anneal" and "an eel," "nitrates" and "night rates," or in "grade A" and "gray day."

This kind of "open" juncture necessarily occurs between sounds. There are also several other kinds of juncture. Consider the pair:

"Her Ladyship awaits without, Seymour."

"Her Ladyship awaits, without Seymour."

The commas in these sentences indicate level juncture, so-called because the voice usually resumes speech, after the gap, at the same level of pitch at which it broke off. The shift of juncture restructures the entire utterance. The word "without," for example, is an adverb in the first sentence but a preposition in the second.

Falling juncture, characterized by rise and fall of pitch, is most commonly the end-signal in a declarative sentence. We hear it after "Seymour" in both examples. Rising juncture, on the other hand, is commonly an end signal in an interrogation such as, "Her Ladyship awaits without, Seymour?" Rising juncture inside an utterance usually separates the elements of a series as in counting: "One, two, three, four . . ." or in listing: "Vanilla, chocolate, strawberry, pistachio . . ."

Pitch, stress, and juncture together provide us with an objective way to distinguish between an incomplete utterance ("I am going . . .") and a complete one ("I am going."). The classic criterion of a "complete thought" is, at best, subjective. But the presence of certain stress-pitch-juncture patterns can be verified simply by speaking or listening.

### It Accentuates the Positive

The structural approach to language has another great advantage: it is positive. The conventional grammar is negative, analyzing utterances only after they have been made, and stamping them, as the Department of Agriculture stamps meat, as acceptable for various levels of users. The structuralist, by contrast, is not trying to teach students to parse sentences that are put before them, but rather to enable them to devise sentences where none existed before.

To this end the chief teaching method is pattern practice. Nearly all English utterances can be reduced to a half-dozen or so basic patterns. One, for example, is the NVN: The boy loves the girl. The dog bites the man. Mantle hit a homer. Such a sentence consists of three parts, but only two different ones, the noun and the verb. These can be expanded into noun clusters and verb clusters. The expansive devices are finite—indeed, very few—but the permutations are infinite.

The noun, for example, grows by an agglutinative process, fore and aft. Single word modifiers come before, in any number but not in any order. The adjective precedes the modifying noun. Thus we say, "The nervous police dog bit the postman," but we do not say, "The police nervous dog bit the postman." From this we can see that the difference between an adjective and a pre-modifying noun is a real one: they pattern differently. We can verify by the simple test of speaking out loud. We can say, "The dilapidated yellow house," or, "The yellow dilapidated house," indifferently. But we cannot reverse the order of the modifiers in "The yellow ranch house."

In the post-modifying position are the adjective phrase and the adjective clause, commonly in that order. Thus, "The nervous police dog in the yard next door who is a friend of mine . . ." All of it is, essentially, an expansion by modification of the single noun, "dog." It can be schematized thus:

| The | nervous | police | dog |
|-----|---------|--------|-----|
| *Determiner* | *Adjective* | *Noun* | *Noun* |

in the yard next door    who is a friend of mine

*Adjective Phrase*      *Adjective Clause*

Abbreviating this, and inserting arrows to show the direction of modification, we arrive at the abstraction:

$$D \quad \rightarrow\!A\!\rightarrow \quad \rightarrow\!N\!\rightarrow \quad N \quad \leftarrow\!AP\!\leftarrow \quad \leftarrow\!ACl\!\leftarrow$$

In the classroom, we might simply begin with that formula and ask the students to flesh it out in real language. Then we can play around with these elements, making elaborate repetitions, substitutions, and expansions. For example, the noun within the adjective phrase can itself become the headword of a noun cluster. Take the phrase "in the front yard" and it can be expanded to "in the weedy, toy-littered front yard of that shiftless Kallikak family that's always disgracing the neighborhood." Students enjoy playing this game. Sometimes the sentences that emerge are shapely and admirable, sometimes not. If not, one can always try again, for the resources of the language are infinite. The point is that the student is learning to use these resources.

Thus, in the NVN, the N's may also be phrases or clauses. Double such a pattern into a parallel construction and you get "To err is human; to forgive, divine." The student comes to such things by stages.

Begin with a simple NVN: "You receive your earnings." Now transform the predicate N into a clause: "You receive what you earn." Now transform into parallel clauses, NCl V NCl "What you receive is what you earn." Now modify the verbs in each clause with a phrase so as to make your reference concrete. "What you receive in happiness is what you have earned in suffering."

The verb expands as well, in its own fashion. The point of this technique is that it is concrete and positive, synthetic rather than analytic. The emphasis is on what you do rather than on what you don't do.

### Talking Prose All His Life

Thus far I have spoken of the bone-structure of language, which the average child has pretty well under control by the age of five. He will add a good deal of vocabulary. And he has yet to learn to read and write, but these are coding processes for the language he already knows.

In theory, he ought to write as fluently as he speaks, once he learns the code. Many teachers ask the student simply to reproduce his speech on paper. He is told to act as his own stenographer, to write it down as he says it. But this advice the student finds astonishingly hard to put into practice. Why?

For one thing, the student does not write as much as he speaks. Who does? He does not even write enough to make the act commonplace. Ideally, he should approach a blank sheet of paper as casually as he sits at a table to eat. But of course he doesn't.

Our students hate to write. It is hate born of fear, for a composition is a deadly game between them and their teacher. Every time the student commits something to paper he incurs the risk of error. Writing at school is a maze of pitfalls—shall or will? Like or as? comma or semicolon? EI or IE? Writing has been taught as an endless series of proscriptions, of things thou shalt *not* do.

The aim of the new grammarians is to convince the student that he has been talking prose all his life, to make him conscious of the linguistic devices he has been using unconsciously. We do not harry him, nag him, and pester him about trivialities of usage.

This does not mean that the linguists have opened the floodgates of illiteracy or have sanctioned the debasement of the tongue of Shakespeare, Milton, and Dwight Macdonald—as has sometimes been charged. This is sheer nonsense derived, I think, from a misunderstanding of the purpose of *descriptive* linguistics, particularly dialect geography. It is a fact that some people say, "He done it. I seen it with my own eyes." Those who chart dialects can tell you who is likely to say this, where, and when. They will not pretend that nobody says it. On the other hand, they will certainly not recommend that if you are given to this kind of speech you apply to NBC for an announcer's job. The linguists supply data, not ethical judgments.

They are aware, too, that "I seen him" is *structurally* no different from "I seed him," "I done seen him," or even, if you insist, "I saw him." None of them can be misunderstood. All of them have the same moral content, which is zero. Once the student realizes that the teacher treats his dialect with the same indifference with which he treats his face, the ground is prepared for learning. The "I seen" speaker attests by his presence in a classroom that he wishes to become an "I saw" speaker. He may not know this, but he can be convinced. Furthermore, you do not attack his problem by picking at his usage errors. Those are the mop-up operations, not the main field of battle. The teacher's basic job is to convince his students that written English is the language he has known all his life; that there is a real relationship, which you can verify and manipulate, between the sounds you make in the air and the marks you put on a paper.

I am all for teaching the dialect of the educated, whatever that may be. But language is different wherever you go, and changing all the time. The material we deal with is alive. As a teacher I advise my student about the current status of linguistic shibboleths, just as the lawyer tells his client where he thinks he may safely chisel on taxes this year. Thus I can tell freshmen that "Who did you see at the party?" is relatively safe by now; but "I seen him" is non-U.

## Don't Blame Miss Prouty

To what extent has structural grammar penetrated the curricula of American schools? The answer is, No more than slightly. On the face of it, this fact is amazing, if not un-American. Characteristically, we are enchanted by the new, contemptuous of yesterday (unless it is nostalgically "antique"). And we are automatically convinced that today's fashions represent Progress. Yet, though my children find my old fountain pen as quaint as a quill, they are still being taught the grammar Thomas Jefferson learned.

Is this because modern linguistics has become so arcane that only a small group of specialists in the graduate schools know what is going on? If so, what can you expect of poor old Miss Prouty, who teaches sixth grade? But Miss Prouty is also teaching the New Mathematics, and relatively up-to-date science. She does not, of course, discourse on genetics and nucleonics in terms remotely like those of the scientists working in these fields. And the new grammar would make no more technical demands on her. So don't blame Miss Prouty.

She is—as a practical matter—subject to the educational Establishment which is dominated by the rebellious generation reared in the so-called Progressive movement of the 1920's and 1930's. The bias of this group is antiacademic, in fact anti-intellectual. Whatever was rigorous, traditional, impractical was anathematized as undemocratic. "Life adjustment" was the objective. "Democratic" education *had* to be good education. Hence the public shock at Sputnik I. The agonizing reappraisal, however, encompassed only mathematics and the sciences—at least at first. It has taken some time for the public to accept the notion (if it has yet) that an illiterate engineer cannot be a good engineer, that a comic-book culture stifles young physicists no less than young novelists.

It was only after huge sums of money, public and private, had been poured into an effort to make a great leap forward in the sciences that the small scattered voices of the humanities began to be heard. Now such enterprises as the federally supported "Project English" are attempting to do for English what has been done already for mathematics, the creation of a sequential modern curriculum from kindergarten to college. At last there is hope of bringing new vitality into our ancient discipline.

But thus far it is hope more than actuality. What is the outlook for the future? In a general way, textbooks are an indicator of classroom practice. A typical case is the 1964 college catalogue of one of the largest textbook publishers in the United States, Scott, Foresman & Company. Listed here under the heading "English Composition" are no less than eighteen composition texts, some of which are used by scores of thousands of students, year after year. Every one of them is traditional in approach. From the technical as distinct from the pedagogical point of view, there is very little choice among them.

In this same catalogue we find—but under a different heading, "English Language"—*A Short Introduction to English Grammar* by the eminent linguist, James Sledd. The author calls his book a "transitional" text, and says in a note to teachers who use the book that "a number of interim textbooks, not one or two, are needed to prepare for some future text which might enjoy a general success in the English classroom." Sledd's book, as he prophesied, has not swept the college field.

Neither have his predecessors', which make a short list. Among these are Lloyd and Warfel, *American English in Its Cultural Setting* (1956); Paul Roberts, *Understanding English* (1958); and the same author's *English Sentences* (1962). Admitting some marginal cases, one could double this catalogue and exhaust it.

For the high school there is Paul Roberts, *Patterns of English,* which is essentially a simpler version of the *Understanding English.* And aimed at the junior high school is Postman, Morine, and Morine, *Discovering Your Language* (1963), a brilliant presentation of modern grammar in a very simple style. It is too soon to know how wide an acceptance this book will have.

When we turn to the lower grades, we find next to nothing. In short, the entry of linguistically oriented grammars into the school system is in the form of an inverted pyramid, with the least where it is needed most.

Like the automobile manufacturers, the textbook houses are Big Business. Both must offer change within continuity. Both must be prepared with some reply to the yearly challenge, "What have you got that's new?" They are too committed to be radical, yet fearful of being left behind. The usual response to this familiar dilemma is compromise. Yet compromise is often impractical, sometimes impossible. You can't design a tight-cornering racing car which is also a gently moving living room for Aunt Tillie. So there is a basic incompatibility between rigorous linguistic analysis and the comfortable old truisms. Nevertheless it is a commonplace now for the publishers to advertise their texts as "structural" or "embodying the best of the new," and so on. The fifth edition of the *Harbrace College Handbook* (1962)—for decades one of the most widely adopted college texts—states in its introduction that "teachers of English composition welcome the new knowledge of grammar that has come from the active linguistic scholarship of the past few decades." For all that, we read in the body of the text that verbs are "indicators of action or a state of being."

The publisher, it seems, is nervously pretending to climb aboard a nonexistent bandwagon without jeopardizing his best sellers. In short, the fraction of our students which is sent to the bookstore to buy a scientific grammar of English is about the same as the fraction of American automobile buyers which purchases all-out sports cars.

Nonetheless I believe it is inevitable that the new will eventually supplant the old, though the change will not be soon or sudden. Several academic generations will be required to teach enough teachers to teach enough teachers—and for enough of those teachers to rise to positions of administrative power where decisions on curricula are made.

## What Makes an Emerson?

And in the meantime there are discouraging difficulties. For instance, the drift of information has been downward, from the graduate school to the grades. Naturally enough, experimental programs and curricular changes have been seeping down in the same direction, despite the fact that the logical way to build a curriculum is from the bottom up.

For three years we conducted a controlled so-called "structural experiment" at the University of Illinois in Chicago. A certain number of sections of freshman rhetoric were taught structural grammar, using the Lloyd-Warfel text, and later the Roberts *Understanding English*. A control group was taught conventionally. Both groups were tested not on their knowledge of grammar, however, but on their improvement in composition. The tests were elaborate and were conducted by disinterested panels of English professors and psychologists. (They of course did not know which group was which.) To the astonishment of some, the two sets of classes came out exactly even. Looked at one way, we didn't do our guinea pigs any harm; from another point of view, we did them no remarkable amount of good.

I was not surprised. I had said at the outset that structural grammar is no panacea; I say it now with authority. If I had it to do over again, I would add a third element to the experiment: a group of students who were taught nothing at all. My prediction is that they would run nose to nose with the others.

We haven't had the nerve to try this experiment, for fear it might put us out of business. My contention is that this has already happened, for we have no more business teaching basic grammar (new or old-fashioned) in colleges than a college mathematics department has teaching the multiplication tables. We never agreed to do it, exactly, but we have taken the job by default. The trouble is that we can't do it. Our students are too old.

We college professors complain that they can't read and write. After a year or more of heroic struggle, we leave them pretty much as we found them. We blame the high schools, the teachers' colleges, our culture—hot rods, TV, comic books, conformity, togetherness—and none of these recriminations teaches a single student how to read and write.

College instructors, at least, have a valid excuse. If they don't teach English composition very well, it is for the excellent reason that they are trying to train the dog after he has grown up. What we have got to do first of all is put grammar back in the grammar school.

At this point I hear the voice of the opposition: "We really taught them in the old days." I agree. A cumbersome and inaccurate system is better than no system at all. In fact, some of those old-fashioned rhetoric teachers did very well indeed.

I am thinking now of Professor Edward Tyrell Channing, who once occupied the chair of Rhetoric at Harvard College. Among his students were R. W. Emerson, Henry Thoreau, James R. Lowell, Edward Everett Hale, Charles Sumner, Oliver Wendell Holmes. . . . He produced some pretty good writers, and he taught them out of Lindley Murray's uncompromisingly Latinical grammar. But Professor Channing did well enough with what he had. Professor Schiller—with all the apparatus of structural linguistics at his disposal—cannot make any comparable claim.

I conclude from this, in all humility, that Professor Channing got a high percentage of Emersons, Thoreaus, and Lowells in his classes, and I do not. Emersons, whether Channing teaches them, or I teach them, turn into Emersons. We can help them sometimes; we probably can't do them too much harm—but we can't make them. They have the language in their bones.

The good student always had sense enough to ignore grammar. His intuition of the language overrode the theory. But what of poor Johnny, who can't read? I'm afraid an occasional reference to a predicate nominative or the subjunctive mood won't help him much. Now that we have undertaken to educate everybody, we need a grammar that really works.

Structural linguistics has given us the tools; we have to learn to use them. In the past few years some of us have brought this theoretical information down to the college freshman level. The next step is the high schools—and we have a very thin end of a wedge in there. But the final objective is the grammar schools. When the day comes that we have finally reinstated grammar—a rational grammar—as a body of subject matter in our elementary schools, on that day we college professors will have reconquered our own territory.

## THE NEW MATH: A PROGRESS REPORT [2]

Debbie, a first-grader, thinks nothing of solving simple equations in alegbra. Everybody in her class does it.

Joe, in the sixth grade, handles problems of logic as well as many college freshmen do.

Are these youngsters geniuses? Their mothers may think so. But actually they are just normal schoolchildren who have been exposed to the new mathematics curriculum.

To most of these youngsters mathematics is a vital, challenging, yet thoroughly understandable subject, rather than the dull drudgery it was for so many people in earlier generations.

The "new math," as it is often called, has stirred up more public interest and curiosity than any other educational reform in this century. Teachers, students, and parents have been drawn into the debate over the merits of modern mathematics, and, in spite of all that has been written and said on the subject, the consensus seems to be that this third of the three R's is certainly far from dull.

Many people still wonder how the "new math" got started, who is responsible for the modern mathematics curriculum, what educators are trying to accomplish with this new curriculum, and most important, whether they have been successful.

In World War II the recruitment of many young men for the armed services revealed shocking inadequacies in their mathe-

[2] From "The Lively Third R," by Kenneth E. Brown, Edwina Deans, and Veryl Schult, all specialists for mathematics at the United States Office of Education, Bureau of Research. *American Education.* 2:9-13. Je. '66. *American Education* is a publication of the United States Office of Education.

matical achievement. By the early 1950's a few scholars who were aware of the weakness of mathematics education in this country were taking steps toward reform. Some had already secured limited financial support for needed experimentation. Among the first to develop a comprehensive program was the University of Illinois Committee on School Mathematics (UICSM), which began experimentation to improve school mathematics curriculum material in 1951.

Some of the initiative for such experimental activities came from individuals, some from professional organizations such as the American Mathematical Society, the Mathematical Association of America, and the National Council of Teachers of Mathematics. These organizations had earlier issued joint reports on the need for curriculum revision, but, in general, these pronouncements fell on deaf ears; the conference reports gathered dust on library shelves.

## Impact of Sputnik

The firing of the first earth satellite, Sputnik I in 1957, is generally considered to be the beginning of the revolution in mathematics education in the United States. This dramatic event made people aware of just how great an explosion of knowledge was taking place in this generation.

The tremendous advances in mathematics research, the increased use of automation, and the widespread introduction of computers helped to emphasize the point Sputnik I had made: Mathematics was of crucial importance; the school mathematics curriculum was obsolete; and reform was badly needed.

After general recognition of the need for curriculum reform, the next step was up to the mathematicians. Throughout the country groups of scholars met to review the needed improvements in the mathematics curriculum. Then, usually in subsequent summers, teams of college teachers, school teachers, and research mathematicians planned course content and wrote sample textbooks. The size of these teams in the various curriculum projects ranged from as few as two or three to as many as forty or fifty.

Many of the ideas in these new materials were tried out in the classroom before they were included in the new curriculum. Writing teams also produced programed textbooks, teachers' guides, enrichment books and pamphlets for students, self-instructional units and tests, correspondence courses, supplementary booklets on applications of mathematics to science, and films.

Much of what the new curriculums contained was not really "new," in the sense of having been recently discovered. In fact, some mathematicians have criticized the use of the term "new math," pointing out that most of the ideas had been discovered by the end of the nineteenth century.

However, if many of the facts contained in modern mathematics courses were not "new," the approach had been changed radically. Modern mathematics curriculums called for new methods of teaching, a revised presentation of the subject, a unified approach to the various areas of mathematics, and a faster pace.

One of the common elements in the new mathematics curriculums is an emphasis on the unifying themes or ideas in mathematics. This emphasis has resulted in bringing rather advanced mathematical concepts into secondary and even elementary school classes. For example, the introduction of the language and concept of sets into the elementary grades has introduced children to symbols and words that are normally reserved for the college student.

The new programs also emphasize the structure of mathematics. Their emphasis is on the basic principles or properties common to many mathematical systems. Previously textbooks tended to treat the characteristics of each mathematical model separately; as a result students learned many seemingly unrelated facts. In the new curriculum students are encouraged to uncover general laws and principles. The approach is that of search and discovery; the goal is an understanding of the *why* as well as the *how*.

Through discovery children often grasp an idea intuitively long before they are ready for the detailed step-by-step analysis of the process. Many teachers have found that children taught by the discovery method get hunches and rapidly formulate ideas which can later be subjected to more formal analysis and proof. The method implies a freedom to make mistakes and to question. It encourages students to use the mathematics they know in finding answers to problems. If the child can answer certain key questions, his teacher can assume that he has a certain depth of understanding even though he cannot express his understanding in words.

### The Abstract and the Concrete

From their earliest school experiences with blocks and puzzles, children work informally with geometric shapes and forms. While geometric lines, points, and planes are abstract ideas, their representations in pictures or in the real environment of the child are concrete. In fact, it is possible that simple concepts of geometry are easier for the child to grasp than much of the abstract work with the operations of addition and subtraction which children have traditionally been expected to master during their first two or three years in school.

Mathematics programs for children of grades 1 to 6 have been greatly enriched and broadened by including some simple algebraic ideas. The mathematical sentence in the form of an equation gives the child a clue to the nature of addition, subtraction, multiplication, and division. The equation lends itself readily to the use of letters or of frames, such as squares, triangles, and ovals as placeholders.

For instance, a child learning addition in a new mathematics course might be given a problem like this: $\triangle + \square = 10$. In solving this simple equation, he would learn that there are many possible replacements for the placeholders, such as $5+5$, $6+4$, $9+1$, and so forth. He also discovers that only a certain set of pairs of numbers makes the equation true: $(0, 10)$, $(1, 9)$, $(2, 8)$, $(3, 7)$, $(4, 6)$, $(5, 5)$.

In the new mathematics curriculums, subtraction and division are presented as the "undoing" of addition and multiplication. Subtraction reverses the action associated with addition. In like manner division reverses the action associated with multiplication.

Children learn that zero is a number having special properties, that it designates "not any," and that when it is added to a number, the same number results: $3+0=3$ or $X + 0 = X$. They also learn that zero is known mathematically as the identity element for addition, because when zero is added to a number the sum is the number itself. They learn that one is the number in multiplication which serves a similar purpose as zero does in addition. It does not change the product: $8 \times 1 = 8$ or $X \times 1 = X$.

Many youngsters in the upper elementary grades and beyond are being introduced to bases of numeration other than ten as one way of helping them gain deeper understanding of our decimal system. This study also helps students develop an appreciation for the way in which base two and base eight are used in the arithmetic of the electronic digital computer.

Some of the new elementary programs are introducing the concepts and terminology of sets. A "set" is a well-defined collection of objects that are not necessarily alike in any way, such as five dimes, six numerals, or four letters of the alphabet. For example, the objects in two sets might consist of a triangle, a square, and a circle; and a balloon, a cart, and a jump rope. In each example there are three things. The objects of one set can be matched one-to-one with the objects of the other. The triangle can be matched with the balloon, the square with the cart, and the circle with the jump rope to show that these are equivalent sets. Both have the same cardinal number, 3. The numeral "3" names the number of objects for either set. The objects in two sets may be combined to make a third set. These procedures of identifying, combining, separating, and comparing when performed with objects or pictured material are roughly analogous to the operations of addition, subtraction, multiplication, and division with numbers.

The new elementary school curriculums emphasize the necessity of children's understanding the values of large and small numbers. More emphasis is placed on estimation and mental arithmetic as essential for the numerical thinking demanded by our society today. The new curriculums also stress the fact that there are different ways of arriving at the same answer.

## Stepping Up the Curriculum

Now that advanced mathematical concepts are being introduced in early grades, mathematics specialists are searching for methods appropriate to the child's level of understanding. For example, early use of the number line has enabled children to progress rapidly from a study of positive whole numbers to the negatives and rationals. Recent programs are emphasizing a laboratory method of teaching mathematics and the individualization of instruction on the elementary school level.

In junior and senior high schools the new mathematics curriculums build upon the foundations of improved elementary training, streamline and combine the traditional high school mathematics courses, and expand old curriculums to include topics which are pertinent to modern needs.

A decade ago the mathematics program in the secondary school quite generally consisted of ninth-grade algebra, tenth-grade geometry, eleventh-grade algebra, and one half year each of trigonometry and solid geometry in the twelfth-grade.

As a result of the 1959 report of the Commission on Mathematics of the College Entrance Examination Board and experimental curriculum projects such as the School Mathematics Study Group's, the program in secondary school mathematics now generally begins with informal geometry including construction and introduction to formal algebra in the seventh grade and concludes with such advanced subjects as probability and statistical inference, matrix algebra, elementary functions, and mathematical analysis in the twelfth grade. A few students may even study the calculus.

Besides the regular mathematics courses, there are many activities which strengthen and enrich the mathematics curriculum in our secondary schools. For example, during the fiscal year 1966 over two thousand high school students of high ability attended special summer training programs sponsored by the National Science Foundation. Mathematics clubs and contests, special lectures and seminars, courses in electronic digital computing, science fairs, and summer mathematics camps encourage students to make individual investigations, motivate them to further study, and help develop their leadership qualities.

The effectiveness of the new secondary school mathematics programs has been questioned almost from the time the new curriculums were first introduced into the high schools. Evaluation has been difficult; a new curriculum necessitated new tests which would measure a student's achievement in the goals of that particular program. Moreover, school administrators, parents, and teachers wanted to be sure that students could do satisfactorily on traditional tests.

As a result, many of the recent research studies on high school mathematics have compared, by means of traditional tests, the achievement of pupils in the new curriculums with those in traditional courses. The traditional tests showed that the pupils in the new programs did learn traditional materials and that they learned materials the other pupils did not have an opportunity to learn.

Other studies are now under way to explore the long-term effects of some of the new mathematics programs. Answers are being sought to such questions as: Have students continued their study of mathematics beyond the required courses? Have they elected mathematics courses in college? Have they pursued scientific careers? How does their college achievement in mathematics compare with students who studied traditional mathematics courses? . . .

As a result of the improved secondary school mathematics curriculums, students are today entering college with better preparation in mathematics than five years ago. Studies indicate that college freshmen are able to take more advanced courses and have a better understanding of the concepts and structures of mathematics. Many high school students are taking advanced placement exams and are getting college credit or placement in sophomore mathematics classes in college. A 1965 survey also reveals that many colleges and universities have significantly revised their freshman year mathematics programs to take into account the better preparation of students for college.

Since many high school dropouts come from the group that is not taking the college preparatory courses, schools are making special efforts to locate or develop new curriculums which will help to motivate the potential dropouts to stay in school until they learn some salable skill.

Various types of "general" mathematics courses are usually offered such students. They are designed to be partly remedial, to give students some new mathematical experiences, to prepare students to solve the problems of their jobs and their daily life, and to strengthen them to enter the college preparatory sequence if they choose to do so.

Numerous groups have prepared curriculum materials for such courses. For instance, the School Mathematics Study Group has rewritten the junior high school mathematics courses to make them more suitable for slower students. The elementary algebra course has been rewritten as a two-year course for students who cannot achieve success in a one-year course. The National Council of Teachers of Mathematics has considered the problem of teaching mathematics to slower students so serious that it has sponsored the writing of units for slow ninth-grade students. The units are being tried out and evaluated in many schools and will be available ... [in the fall of 1966].

## *Value of the Laboratory*

The "why" approach has been found to help the casual students as much as it does the student who has a particular talent for mathematics. This approach can often be taught best through the use of learning aids. Under the National Defense Education Act of 1958, the Office of Education administers a program through which Federal grants are made to state educational agencies to aid local public schools in acquiring specialized equipment and materials for strengthening instruction in mathematics and eight other critical subjects. During the first seven years of this program state or local educational agencies have matched over $30 million in Federal funds for the purchase of instructional equipment in the field of mathematics. These devices have run the gamut from number line aids to electronic computers and have included such items as reference books, counting frames, geometric models, calculators, aids for explaining fundamental operations, area and volume measurement devices, and overhead projectors.

These instructional aids have enabled many teachers to utilize more than ever before a laboratory or discovery approach. It is estimated that there are currently two thousand well-equipped mathematics laboratories in the United States.

The laboratory gives pupils at all levels of ability a chance to explore and discover mathematics under the guidance of a well-qualified mathematics teacher. It stimulates the able child, opens new avenues of experience for him, and encourages him to progress as rapidly as he is able. The slow student profits from the learning aids the laboratory provides as they make it possible for him to work at his own pace in reaching abstract levels of thinking.

Along with the curriculum reforms and increased use of learning aids came a need for teacher training and retraining. Teachers who had fulfilled all the requirements for certification only a few years earlier found themselves unprepared to cope with the "new math." College training for future mathematics teachers had to be improved and in-service training programs for those already teaching had to be set up to insure that teachers would put the new curriculums to the best possible use.

In the last decade America has seen the largest "back to school" movement by teachers ever witnessed. The newer aspects of arithmetic, algebra, geometry, and analysis are still being taught in thousands of classes held on Saturdays, after school hours, and during holidays.

In order to update the undergraduate training of mathematics teachers, organizations such as the Mathematical Association of America have set up special committees to develop broad programs of improvement in college and university curriculums. Such committees have also drawn up recommendations of minimum standards for the training of teachers at all levels.

Many types of in-service education programs have been established for teachers who have found that the new curriculums call for a broader and deeper knowledge of mathematics than they possess. Teachers are filling their needs in countless ways, ranging from individual reading to sabbatical leave for a full academic year of study at a college or university.

Mathematics consultants or supervisors at the state level have sponsored widespread in-service training in a systematic effort to provide the opportunity for every elementary and secondary school teacher to upgrade his teaching competence. Local school systems have also sponsored in-service work which is planned especially for the particular system.

## Keeping Teachers Abreast

The urgency of the need for the continuing education of mathematics teachers has led the National Science Foundation (NSF) to provide summer and in-service institutes for elementary, secondary, and college teachers and supervisors. For secondary school personnel it also provides academic year institutes, opportunities to participate in research, and cooperative college-school science programs. In 1966 about 36,000 teachers will study in these various programs. More than $100 million in Federal funds has been spent in NSF mathematics institutes for secondary school teachers alone.

The continuing education of teachers is one of the most important factors in insuring that the new mathematics curriculums are put to the best possible use. Before new mathematics programs can be introduced successfully into our school systems, it is also necessary for superintendents, principals, and other administrators to become informed about new programs and convinced of their worth. In order to meet this need, regional conferences have been held throughout the country. These provided opportunities for participants to become informed or to share their knowledge of ways and means of improving their mathematics programs.

Local school districts have extended such opportunities for discussion of and inquiry into the "new math" to cities and counties. Various professional organizations have highlighted new mathematics programs at their meetings and in their journals in a concentrated effort to reach all persons in positions of leadership. The National Council of Teachers of Mathematics has prepared a film, "Mathematics for Tomorrow," which has been widely circulated in all sections of the country.

State departments of education and local school systems have also prepared bulletins and leaflets to provide information. Courses in the new mathematics have been offered for interested parents. In one city the demand for such courses was so great that it was necessary to hold more than thirty such courses in a single year, with about fifty parents in each. Television programs have informed the public about new developments in mathematics and have tried to give parents some insight into the content of new programs. Publishers have prepared textbooks for parents, and magazines have run numerous articles on new trends in mathematics education. Even though much has been done to inform the public, the Office of Education still receives many questions about the new mathematics, some of which we have tried to answer here.

In spite of all that still needs to be done to bring the teaching of mathematics in this country up to a high level of excellence, we have come a great deal closer to this goal in only a few years. Since the time when Sputnik first circled the globe, a revolution has occurred, and a new, up-to-date curriculum has taken root in our mathematics classrooms.

## APPLYING THE NEW TECHNOLOGY [3]

"Public education is the last great stronghold of the manual trades," John Henry Martin, superintendent of schools in Mount Vernon, New York, recently told a congressional committee. "In education, the industrial revolution has scarcely begun."

But begun it has—slowly, to be sure, but irresistibly, and with the most profound consequences for both education and industry. The past year has seen an explosion of interest in the application of electronic technology to education and training. Hardly a week or month goes by without an announcement from some electronics manufacturer or publishing firm that it is entering the "education market" via merger, acquisition, joint venture, or working arrangement. . . . And a number of electronics firms have been building substantial capabilities of their own in the education field.

[3] From "Technology Is Knocking at the Schoolhouse Door," by Charles E. Silberman, staff writer. *Fortune.* 74:120-5+. Ag '66. Reprinted from the August 1966 issue of Fortune Magazine by special permission; © 1966 Time Inc.

Business has discovered the schools, and neither is likely to be the same again. It may be a bit premature to suggest, as Superintendent Martin does, that "the center of gravity for educational change is moving from the teachers' college and the superintendent's office to the corporation executive suite." But there can be no doubt about the long-term significance of business' new interest in the education market. The companies now coming into the market have resources—of manpower and talent as well as of capital—far greater than the education market has ever seen before. They have, in addition, a commitment to innovation and an experience in management that is also new to the field.

The romance between business and the schools began when the Federal Government took on the role of matchmaker. Indeed, the new business interest in education is a prime example of Lyndon Johnson's "creative federalism" at work. Federal purchasing power is being used to create—indeed, almost to invent—a sizable market for new educational materials and technologies. Until now, the stimulus has come mainly from the Department of Defense and the Office of Economic Opportunity. But the Elementary and Secondary Education Act of 1965 provided large Federal grants to the schools for the purchase of textbooks, library books, audio-visual equipment, etc. It also greatly expanded the Office of Education's research-and-development activities and gave it the prerogative, for the first time, to contract with profit-making as well as nonprofit institutions.

## Computerized Teaching

The most remarkable characteristic of industry's invasion of the education market is that it has been accompanied by the affiliation of otherwise unrelated businesses. The electronics companies have felt the need for "software," i.e., organized informational and educational material, to put into their equipment and have gone in search of such publishing companies as possessed it. Some of the publishing companies, in turn, particularly textbook publishers, have been apprehensive about the long-range future of their media and willingly joined in such auspicious marriages of convenience. As RCA's Chairman David Sarnoff explained his company's merger with Random House last May, "They have the software and we have the hardware."

The fact is that, as far as education is concerned, neither side has either—yet. In time, the application of electronic technology can and will substantially improve the quality of instruction. Experiments with the Edison Responsive Environment Talking Typewriter . . . suggest that it has great potential for teaching children to read. IBM has been working on the development of teaching systems since the late 1950's and is now selling its "IBM 1500 instructional system" to a limited number of educators for research, development, and operational use. But a lot of problems—in hardware as well as software—will have to be solved before the computer finds wide acceptance as a teaching device. No computer manufacturer, for example, has begun to solve the technical problems inherent in building a computer that can respond to spoken orders or correct an essay written in natural language and containing a normal quota of misspellings and grammatical errors—and none has promised it can produce machines at a cost that can compete with conventional modes of instruction.

On the other hand, without the appropriate software, a computerized teaching system results in what computer people call a "GIGO system"—garbage in and garbage out. "The potential value of computer-assisted instruction," as Dr. Launor F. Carter, senior vice president of System Development Corporation, flatly states, "depends on the quality of the instructional material" that goes into it. But the software for a computer-assisted instructional system does not yet exist; indeed, no one yet knows how to go about producing it. The new "education technology industry," as Professor J. Sterling Livingston of Harvard Business School pointed out at a Defense Department-Office of Education conference in June, "is not being built on any important technology of its own." On the contrary, it "is being built as a satellite of the information technology industry. It is being built on the technology of information processing, storage, retrieval, transmission, and reduction . . . by firms whose primary objective is that of supplying information processing and reproduction equipment and services." And neither these firms, nor the professional educators, nor the scholars studying the learning process know enough about how people learn or how they can be taught to use the computers effectively.

### Discovering the Questions to Be Asked

That knowledge is now being developed. The attempts at computer application have dramatized the degree of our ignorance, because the computer, in order to be programed, demands a precision of knowledge about the processes of learning and teaching that the human teacher manages to do without. So far, therefore, the main impact of the computer has been to force a great many people from a great many different disciplines to study the teaching process; they are just beginning to discover what questions have to be asked to develop the theories of learning and of instruction they need.

In time, to be sure, both the hardware and the software problems will be solved, and when they are, the payoff may be large. It will come, however, only to those able to stay the course. And the course will be hard and long—five years, under the most optimistic estimate, and more probably ten or fifteen years. Anyone looking for quick or easy profits would be well advised to drop out now. Indeed, the greatest fear firms like IBM and Xerox express is not that someone may beat them to the market, but that some competitor may rush to market too soon and thereby discredit the whole approach. A number of firms—several with distinguished reputations —did precisely that five years or so ago when they offered shoddy programs to the schools and peddled educationally worthless "teaching machines" and texts door to door.

A lot more is at stake, needless to say, than the fortunes of a few dozen corporations, however large. The new business-government thrust in education, with its apparent commitment to the application of new technologies, is already changing the terms of the debate about the future of American education, creating new options and with them, new priorities. "We have been dealt a new set of cards," Theodore R. Sizer, dean of Harvard's Graduate School of Education, has remarked, "and we must learn how to play with them."

Rarely have U.S. corporations assumed a role so fraught with danger for the society, as well as for themselves, or so filled with responsibility and opportunity. For over the long run, the new business-government thrust is likely to transform both the organization and the content of education, and through it, the character and shape of American society itself. And the timing could not be more propitious. It is already clear that we have barely scratched the surface of man's ability to learn, and there is reason to think that we may be on the verge of a quantum jump in learning and in man's creative use of intellect. Certainly the schools and colleges are caught up in a ferment as great as any experienced since the great experiment of universal education began a century or so ago. Every aspect of education is subject to change: the curriculum, the instruments of education, the techniques and technology of instruction, the organization of the school, the philosophy and goals of education. And every stage and kind of education is bound up in change: nursery schools; elementary and secondary schools, both public and private, secular and parochial; colleges and universities; adult education; vocational training and rehabilitation.

### Failure in the Ghetto and the Suburb

The schools have been in ferment since the postwar era began, with the pace of change accelerating since the early and middle 1950's. Until fairly recently they were so deluged with the sheer problem of quantity—providing enough teachers, classrooms, textbooks to cope with the numbers of students that had to be admitted —that they had little energy for, or interest in, anything else. And now the pressure of numbers is hitting the high schools and colleges.

It is becoming clearer and clearer, however, that dealing with quantity is the least of it: most of the problems and most of the opportunities confronting the schools grow out of the need for a broad overhaul of public education. For more than a decade, a small band of reformers—among them Jerome Bruner, Jerrold Zacharias, Francis Keppel, John Gardner, Lawrence Cremin, Francis Ianni—have been engaged in an heroic effort to lift the quality and change the direction of public education. Their goal has been to create something the world has never seen and previous generations could not even have imagined: a mass educational system successfully dedicated to the pursuit of intellectual excellence. . . .

This effort at reform has two main roots. The first, and in many ways most important, has been the recognition—largely forced by the civil rights movement—that the public schools were failing to provide any sort of education worthy of the name to an intolerably large segment of the population. This failure is not diffused evenly throughout the society; it is concentrated in the rural and urban slums and racial ghettos. The failure is not new; as Lawrence Cremin and others have demonstrated, public education has *always* had a strong class bias in the United States, and it has never been as universal or as successful as we have liked to believe. But in the contemporary world the schools' failure to educate a large proportion of its students has become socially and morally intolerable.

At the same time there has been a growing realization that the schools are failing white middle-class children, too—that all children, white as well as black, "advantaged" as well as "disadvantaged," can and indeed must learn vastly more than they are now being taught. By the early 1950's it had become apparent that even in the most privileged suburbs the schools were not teaching enough, and that they were teaching the wrong things and leaving out the right things. Where the schools fell down most abysmally was in their inability to develop a love for learning and their failure to teach youngsters how to learn, to teach them independence of thought, and to train them in the uses of intuition and imagination.

The remaking of American education has taken a number of forms. The most important, by far, has been the drive to reform the curriculum—in Jerrold Zacharias' metaphor, to supply the schools with "great compositions"—i.e., new courses, complete with texts, films, laboratory equipment, and the like, created by the nation's leading scholars and educators. This has *not* meant a return to *McGuffey's Reader* or the "Great Books," however. Quite the contrary; the "explosion of knowledge," combined with its instant dissemination, has utterly destroyed the old conception of school as the place where a person accumulates most of the knowledge he will need over his lifetime. Much of the knowledge today's students will need hasn't been discovered yet, and much of what is now being taught is (or may soon become) obsolete or irrelevant.

What students need most, therefore, is not more information but greater depth of understanding, and greater ability to apply that understanding to new situations as they arise. "A merely well-informed man," that greatest of modern philosophers, the late Alfred North Whitehead, wrote forty-odd years ago, "is the most useless bore on God's earth." Hence the aim of education must be "the acquisition of the art of the utilization of knowledge."

## Reforming the Teachers

It has become increasingly apparent, however, that reform of the curriculum, crucial as it is, is too small a peg on which to hang the overhaul of the public school. For one thing, the reformers have found that it is a good deal harder to "get the subject right" than they had ever anticipated. And getting it right doesn't necessarily get it adopted or well taught. Five years ago Professor Zacharias was confident that with $100 million a year for new courses, texts, films, and the like he could work a revolution in the quality of U.S. education. Now he's less confident. "It's easier to put a man on the moon," he says, "than to reform the public schools."

Reform is impeded by the professional educators themselves, whose inertia can hardly be imagined by anyone outside the schools, as well as by the anti-intellectualism of a public more interested in athletics than in the cultivation of the mind. The most important bar to change, however, is the fact that the new curricula, and in particular the new teaching methods, demand so much more of teachers than they can deliver. Some teachers are unwilling to adopt the new courses; the majority simply lack the mastery of subject matter and of approach that the new courses require.

It does no good to reform the curriculum, therefore, without reforming the teachers, and, indeed, the whole process of instruction. Under present methods this process is grossly inefficient. One reason is that so few attempts have been made to improve it in any fundamental way. Without question, the schools would be greatly improved if, as James Bryant Conant and others have suggested, they could attract and retain more teachers who know and like their subjects and who also like to teach. A great deal has been accomplished along these lines in recent years, and the experience suggests some kind of reversal of Gresham's Law: raising standards seems to attract abler people into the teaching profession. But something more is needed: teachers have to know how to teach—how to teach hostile or unmotivated children as well as the highly motivated. Until recently, however, most of the creative people concerned with education have been convinced that teaching is an art which a person either has or lacks, and which in any case defies precise description. Hence their failure to study the process of instruction in any scientific or systematic way. (The collection of banalities, trivialities, and misinformation that make up most of the courses in "method" in most teachers' colleges represents the antithesis of this kind of study.)

### Organized to Prevent Learning

To be sure, teaching—like the practice of medicine—is very much an art, which is to say, it calls for the exercise of talent and creativity. But like medicine, it is also—or should be—a science, for it involves a repertoire of techniques, procedures, and skills that can be systematically studied and described, and therefore transmitted and improved. The great teacher, like the great doctor, is the one who adds creativity and inspiration to that basic repertoire. In large measure, the new interest in the development of electronic teaching technologies stems from the growing conviction that the process of instruction, no less than the process of learning, is in fact susceptible to systematic study and improvement.

Part of the problem, moreover, is that most of the studies of the teaching process that have been conducted until fairly recently have ignored what goes on in the classroom, excluding as "extraneous" such factors as the way the classroom or the school is organized. Yet it is overwhelmingly clear that one of the principal reasons children do not learn is that the schools are organized to facilitate administration rather than learning—to make it easier for teachers and principals to maintain order rather than to make it easier for children to learn. Indeed, to a degree that we are just beginning to appreciate as the result of the writings of such critics as Edgar Z. Friedenberg, John Holt, and Bel Kaufman, schools and classrooms are organized so as to *prevent* learning or teaching from taking place.

## The New Concept of Intelligence

The solution, however, is not, as impatient (and essentially anti-intellectual) romanticists like Paul Goodman and John Holt seem to advocate, to abolish schools—i.e., to remove the "artificial" institutions and practices we seem to put between the child and his innate desire to learn. To be sure, the most remarkable feat of learning any human ever performs—learning to speak his native tongue —is accomplished, in the main, without any formal instruction. But while every family talks, *no* family possesses more than a fraction of the knowledge the child must acquire in addition. It would be insane to insist that every child discover that knowledge for himself; the transmission of knowledge—new as well as old—has always been regarded as one of the distinguishing characteristics of human society; and that means, quite simply, that man cannot depend upon a casual process of learning; he must be "educated."

He not only must be educated; he *can* be educated—of this there no longer can be any doubt. The studies of the learning process conducted over the past twenty years have made it abundantly clear that those who are not now learning properly—say, the bottom 30 to 50 per cent of the public-school population—can in fact learn, and can learn a great deal, if they are properly taught from the beginning. (These studies make it equally clear that those who *are* learning can learn vastly more.) This proposition grows out of the repudiation of the old concept of fixed or "native" intelligence and its replacement by a new concept of intelligence as something that is itself learned. To be sure, nature does set limits of sorts. But they are very wide limits; precisely what part of his genetic potential an individual uses is determined in good measure by his environment, which is to say, by his experiences.

And the most important experiences are those of early child-hood. The richer the experience in these early years, the greater the development of intelligence. As the great Swiss child psychologist Jean Piaget puts it, "the more a child has seen and heard, the more he wants to see and hear." And the less he has seen and heard, the less he wants—and is able—to see and hear and understand. Hence the growing emphasis on preschool education.

The abandonment of the concept of fixed intelligence requires changes all along the line. The most fundamental is a new concern for individual differences, which Professor Patrick Suppes of Stanford calls "the most important principle of learning as yet unaccepted in the working practice of classroom and subject-matter teaching." To be sure, educators have been talking about the need to take account of individual differences in learning for at least forty years—but for forty years they've been doing virtually nothing about it, in large part because they have lacked both the pedagogy and the technology.

Now, however, the technology is becoming available—and at a time when there is a growing insistence that the schools *must* take account of individual differences. Indeed, this quest for ways to individualize instruction is emerging as the most important single force for innovation and reform.

In part, the demand grows out of recent research on learning, which has made it clear, as Professor Susan Meyer Markle of UCLA has put it, that "individualized instruction is a necessity, not a luxury." In part, too, the demand stems from the conviction, as Lawrence Cremin puts it, that "any system of universal education is ultimately tested at its margins"—by its ability to educate gifted and handicapped as well as "average" youngsters.

The pressure for individualization of instruction is developing even more strongly as a byproduct of the efforts at desegregation of the public schools. Because of the schools'—and society's—past failures, Negro children tend to perform below the level of the white students with whom they are mingled. They need a lot of special attention and help in order to overcome past deficits and fulfill their own potential. Few schools are providing this help; most educators are simply overwhelmed by problems for which their training and experience offer no guide. And so they tend to deal with the problem in one of two ways: by ignoring it (in which case either the Negro or the white students, or both, are shortchanged); or by putting the children into homogeneous "ability groups," in which case they are simply resegregated according to IQ or standardized test scores. Neither approach is likely to be acceptable for very long. The need is for a system of instruction in which all students are seen as special students, and in which, in Lyndon Johnson's formulation, each is offered all the education that his or her ambition demands and that his or her ability permits.

## Corn for the Behaving Pigeon

Enter the computer! What makes it a potentially important—perhaps revolutionary—educational instrument is precisely the fact that it offers a technology by which, for the first time, instruction really *can* be geared to the specific abilities, needs, and progress of each individual.

The problem is how. Most of the experimentation with computer-assisted instruction now going on is based, one way or another, on the technique of "programed instruction" developed in the 1950's by a number of behavioral psychologists, most notably B. F. Skinner of Harvard. Professor Skinner defines learning as a change in behavior, and the essence of his approach is his conviction that any behavior can be produced in any person by "reinforcing," i.e., rewarding closer and closer approximations to it. It is immaterial what reward is used: food (corn for a pigeon, on which most of Skinner's experiments have been conducted, or candy for a child), praise, or simply the satisfaction a human being derives from knowing he is right. What is crucial is simply that the desired behavior be appropriately rewarded—and that it be rewarded right away. By using frequent reinforcement of small steps, the theory holds, one can shape any student's behavior toward any predetermined goal.

To teach a body of material in this way, it is necessary first to define the goal in precise and measurable terms—a task educators normally duck. Then the material must be broken down into a series of small steps—thirty to one hundred frames per hour of instruction—and presented in sequence. As a rule, each sequence, or frame, consists of one or more statements, followed by a question the student must answer correctly before proceeding to the next frame. Since the student checks his own answer, the questions necessarily are in a form that can be answered briefly, e.g., by filling in a word, indicating whether a statement is true or false, or by choosing which of, say, four answers is correct. (Most programers have abandoned the use of "teaching machines," which were simply devices for uncovering the answer and advancing to the next frame. Programs are now usually presented in book form, with answers in a separate column in the margin; the student covers the answers with a ruler or similar device, which he slides down the page as needed.) If the material has been programed correctly—so the theory holds— every student will be able to master it, though some will master it faster than others. If anyone fails to learn, it is the fault of the program, not of the student. Programed instruction, in short, is a teaching technology that purports to be able to teach every student, and at his own pace.

But teach him what? That's the rub. Most of the applications of programed instruction have been in training courses for industry and the armed forces, where it is relatively easy to define the knowledge or skills to be taught in precise behavioral terms, and where the motivation to learn is quite strong. (One survey of industry's use of programed instruction indicated that 69 per cent of the programs used were "job-oriented.") It's a lot harder to specify the "behavior" to be produced, say, by a course in Shakespeare or in American history, and a lot more difficult to sustain the interest of a student whose job or rank does not depend directly on how well he learns the material at hand. And the small steps and the rigidity of the form of presentation and the limitation of response make a degree of boredom inevitable, at least for students with some imagination and creativity.

If programing is used too extensively, moreover, it may prevent the development of intuitive and creative thinking or destroy such thinking when it appears. For one thing, programing instruction seems to force a student into a relatively passive role, whereas most learning theorists agree that no one can really master a concept unless he is forced to express it in his own words or actions and to construct his own applications and examples. It is not yet clear, however, whether this defect is inherent in the concept of programing or is simply a function of its present primitive state of development. A number of researchers are trying to develop programs that present material through sound and pictures as well as print, and require students to give an active response in a variety of ways— e.g., drawing pictures or diagrams, writing whole sentences. Donald Cook, manager of the Xerox education division's applied-research department, has experimented with programs to teach students how to listen to a symphony. And Professor Richard Crutchfield of the University of California at Berkeley is using programed instruction techniques to try to teach students how to think creatively—how to construct hypotheses, how to use intelligent guessing to check the relevance of the hypotheses, etc.

## Teaching by Discovery

More important, perhaps, the rigidity of structure that seems to be inherent in programed instruction may imply to students that there is indeed only one approach, one answer; yet what the students may need to learn most is that some questions may have more than one answer or no answer at all. Programed instruction would appear to be antithetical to the "discovery method" favored by Bruner, Zacharias, and most of the curriculum reformers. This is a technique of inductive teaching through which students discover the fundamental principles and structures of each subject for themselves. Instead of telling students why the American colonists revolted against George III, for example, a history teacher using "the discovery method" would give them a collection of documents from the period and ask them to find the causes themselves.

The conflict between programed instruction and the discovery method may be more apparent than real. At the heart of both (as well as of the "Montessori method") is a conception of instruction as something teachers do *for* students rather than *to* them, for all three methods approach instruction by trying to create an environment that students can manipulate for themselves. The environment may be the step-by-step presentation of information through programed instruction; it may be the source documents on the American revolution that students are asked to read and analyze, but that someone first had to select, arrange, and try out; it may be the assortment of blocks, beads, letters, numbers, etc., of the Montessori kindergarten.

There is general agreement, however, that at the moment, programed instruction can play only a limited role in the schools. Apart from anything else, it is enormously expensive; the cost of constructing a good program runs from $2,000 to $6,000 per student-hour. Because of the costs and the primitive state of the art, Donald Cook believes it inadvisable to try to program an entire school course; programing should be reserved for units of five to fifteen hours of work, teaching specific sets of information or skills that can (or must) be presented in sequence (e.g., multiplication tables or rules of grammar) and whose mastery, as he puts it, offers "a big payoff." In this way teachers can be relieved of much of the drill that occupies so much classroom time; if students can come to class having mastered certain basic information and skills, teachers and students can conduct class discussions on a much higher level.

When the proper limitations are observed, therefore, programed instruction can be enormously useful, both as a means of individualizing instruction and as a research instrument that can lead to greater understanding of the learning and the teaching processes. It is being used in both these ways at the Oakleaf School in Whitehall, Pennsylvania, just outside Pittsburgh . . . where the most elaborate experiment in the development of a system of individualized instruction is being carried out under the direction of Professors Robert Glaser, John Bolvin, and C. M. Lindvall of the University of Pittsburgh's Learning Research and Development Center.

## The Uses of Feedback

Computers and their associated electronic gadgetry offer ways of remedying some of the obvious defects of programed instruction. For example, programs generally involve only one sense—sight—

whereas most learning theorists believe that students learn faster and more easily if *several* senses are brought into play. Electronic technology makes it possible to do just that. When a youngster presses one of the keys on the Edison Responsive Environment's Talking Typewriter, the letter appears in print in front of him, while a voice tells him the name of it. When he has learned the alphabet, the machine will tell him—aurally—to type a word; the machine can be programed so that the student can depress only the correct keys, in correct order. And at Patrick Suppes' Computer-Based Mathematics Laboratory at Stanford University . . . students using earlier versions of IBM's new 1500 Computer-Assisted Instructional System receive instructions or information aurally (through prerecorded sound messages) or visually (through photographs, diagrams, or words and sentences that are either projected on a cathode-ray tube or presented in conventional typewritten form). Students may respond by typing the answer, by writing on the cathode-ray tube with an electronic "light pen," or by pushing one of several multiple-choice buttons.

To be sure, the 1500 system is still experimental—wide commercial application is five years away—and much richer and far more flexible "environments" are necessary to make the computer a useful teaching device. But computer manufacturers are confident that they can come up with wholly new kinds of input and output devices.

What makes the computer so exciting—and potentially so significant—is its most characteristic attribute, feedback, i.e., its ability to modify its own operation on the basis of the information fed into it. It is this that opens up the possibility of responding to each student's performance by modifying the curriculum as he goes along. This couldn't be done now. Programed instruction currently deals with individual differences in a crude way, chiefly by permitting students to move along as slowly or as rapidly as they can; they still all deal essentially with the same material. But speed of learning is only one relevant dimension of individual differences, and not necessarily the most important. Suppes, among others, is convinced that the best way to improve learning is through "an almost single-minded concentration on individual differences" in the way material is presented to the student.

What this means, in practice, is that a teacher should have a number of different programs at his disposal, since no single strategy of instruction or mode of presentation is likely to work for every student. Second, he should be able to select the most appropriate program for each student on the basis of that student's current knowledge, past performance, and personality. Third and most important, he should be able to modify the program for each student as he goes along in accordance with what the student knows and doesn't know, the kinds of materials he finds difficult and the kinds he learns easily. In time it should be practicable to program a computer to assist in all of these functions.

### Games Students Play

Computers lend themselves to the "discovery method" as well as to programed instruction. The exercise of simulating situations and playing games on a computer, for example, can help a student gain insight into a problem by making it possible for him to experiment—and to see the consequences of his (or other people's) actions in much shorter time than is possible in real life. The computer also imposes a strong discipline on the student, forcing him to analyze a problem in a logically consistent manner, while freeing him from a good deal of time-consuming computation.

The armed forces have been using computer simulation and computer games to teach military strategy, and the American Management Association to teach business strategy. Now, a number of researchers, among them Professor James Coleman of Johns Hopkins, are trying to adapt the technique to the instruction of high school students. Preliminary results suggest that it may be particularly effective in teaching the so-called "disadvantaged" and "slow learners," whose motivation to learn in ordinary classroom situations has been destroyed by years of failure.

As with computer-assisted programed instruction, costs will have to come down dramatically, and techniques for addressing the computer in natural language will have to be developed before widespread application is possible. In the meantime the experiments with computer games have led a number of educational researchers to try to develop nonmechanical games of the Monopoly variety for teaching purposes, especially in the social sciences.

Computers are likely to enhance learning in still another way —by increasing both the amount of information students have at their disposal and the speed with which they can get it. In time electronic storage, retrieval, and presentation of information should make it possible for students or scholars working in their local library—ultimately, perhaps, in their own home—to have access to all the books and documents in all the major libraries around the country or the world. A great many technical problems remain to be solved, however, as everyone working on information retrieval knows through hard (and sometimes bitter) experience.

### Thoughts in a Marrow Bone

The biggest obstacle to the introduction of computer-assisted instruction is not technological; it is our ignorance about the process of instruction. Significant progress has been made, however, in identifying what needs to be known before a theory of instruction can be developed. It is clear, for example, that any useful theory must explain the role of language in learning and teaching—including its role in *preventing* learning. It is language, more than anything else, that distinguishes human from animal learning; only man can deal with the world symbolically and linguistically. But verbalization is not the only way people learn or know, as Jerome Bruner of Harvard emphasizes. We know things "enactively," which is to say, in our muscles. Children can be very skillful on a seesaw without having any concept of what it is and without being able to represent it by drawing a balance beam (the use of imagery) or by writing Newton's law of moments (symbolic representation). Present teaching methods, Bruner argues, place too much emphasis on the verbal—a fact he likes to illustrate by quoting these magnificent lines from Yeats:

> God guard me from those thoughts men think
> In the mind alone;
> He that sings a lasting song
> Thinks in a marrow-bone

The result is that youngsters too often display great skill in using words that describe words that describe words, with no real feel for, or image of, the concrete phenomenon itself.

Knowing something, moreover, involves at least two distinct processes. The first is memory, the ability to recall the information or concept on demand; and the second is what learning theorists call "transfer," i.e., the ability not only to retrieve the knowledge that is in the memory but to apply it to a problem or situation that differs from the one in which the information was first acquired. We know somewhat more about memory, and recent discoveries in molecular biology hold the promise of vast gains in our understanding of it and our ability to improve it. . . .

Most learning theorists, however, believe that transfer is more important than memory, and that the degree of transfer a student develops depends on how, as well as what, he was taught. For transfer involves a number of specific and distinct traits or skills. A person must be able to recognize when a problem is present. He must be able to arrange problems in patterns—to see that each problem is not entirely unique but has at least some elements in common with other problems he has solved in the past. He must have sufficient internal motivation to want to solve the problem, and enough self-discipline to persist in the face of error. He must know how to ask questions and generate hypotheses, and how to use guessing and first approximations to home in on the answer. There is reason to think that these skills can be taught. In any case, we must know far more than we do now about both memory and transfer before we can develop the theory of instruction needed to program computers effectively.

Besides that, we need to know more about how the way material is presented—for example, the sequence, size of steps, order of words—affects learning. And we need to understand how to make children—all children—*want* to learn. We need to know how to make children coming from "intellectually advantaged" as well as "disadvantaged" homes regard school learning as desirable and pleasurable. The problem is larger than it may seem, for there is a deep strain of anti-intellectualism running through American life. The notion that intellectual activity is effete and effeminate takes hold among the boys around the fifth grade, and becomes both deep and widespread in the junior high years, when youngsters are most susceptible to pressure from their peers. (Curiously enough, the notion that intellectual activity is *un*feminine sets in among girls at about the same age.) We need to know how to overcome these widespread cultural attitudes, as well as the emotional and neurological "blocks" that prevent some youngsters from learning at all. And we must understand far better than we now do how different kinds of rewards and punishments affect learning.

Interestingly enough, one of the greatest advantages the computer possesses may well be its impersonality—the fact that it can exhibit infinite patience in the face of error without registering disappointment or disapproval—something no human teacher can ever manage. These qualities may make a machine superior to a teacher in dealing with students who have had a record of academic failure, whether through organic retardation, emotional disturbance, or garden-variety learning blocks. The impersonality of the machine may be useful for average or above-average children as well, since it increases the likelihood that a youngster may decide to learn to please himself rather than to please his parents or teachers. And motivation must become "intrinsic" rather than "extrinsic" if children are to develop their full intellectual capacity.

There is reason to think that we may need a number of theories of learning and instruction. For one thing, the process of learning probably differs according to what it is that is being learned. As the Physical Science Study Committee put it in one of its annual reports, "We have all but forgotten, in recent years, that the verb 'to learn' is transitive; there must be some thing or things that the student learns." Unless that thing seems relevant to a student, he will have little interest in learning it (and he will derive little or no reward from its mastery). In any case, different subjects—or different kinds of students—may require different methods of instruction; a method that works wonderfully well in teaching physics may not work in teaching the social sciences.

More important, perhaps, different kinds of students may require different teaching strategies. It is only too evident that methods that work well with brighter-than-average upper-middle-class families fail dismally when used with children, bright or dull, from a city or rural slum. And differences in income and class are not the only variables; a student's age, sex, ethnic group, and cultural background all affect the way his mind operates as well as his attitude toward learning. Differences in "cognitive style" may also have to be taken into account—for example, the fact that some people have to see something to understand it, while others seem to learn more easily if they hear it.

## *What Knowledge Is Worth Most?*

When adequate theories of instruction have been developed, the new educational-system designers will still have to decide what it is that they want to teach. That decision cannot be made apart from the most fundamental decisions about values and purpose—the values of the society as well as the purpose of education. What we teach reflects, consciously or unconsciously, our concept of the good life, the good man, and the good society. Hence "there is no avoiding the question of purpose," as Laurence Cremin insists. And given the limited time children spend in school and the growing influence of other educational agencies, there is no avoiding the question of priorities—deciding what knowledge is of most worth.

The answers will be very much affected by the new electronic technologies. Indeed, the computer will probably force a radical reappraisal of educational content as well as educational method, just as the introduction of the printed book did. When knowledge could be stored in books, the amount of information that had to be stored in the human brain (which is to say, committed to memory) was vastly reduced. The "antitechnologists" of antiquity were convinced that the book, by downgrading memory, could produce only a race of imbeciles.

This discovery of yours [Socrates told the inventor of the alphabet in the *Phaedrus*], will create forgetfulness in the learners' souls, because they will not use their memories; they will trust to the external written characters and not remember of themselves. . . . They will appear to be omniscient and will generally know nothing.

The computer will enormously increase the amount of information that can be stored in readily accessible form, thereby reducing once again the amount that has to be committed to memory. It will also drastically alter the role of the teacher. But it will not replace him; as some teaching-machine advocates put it, any teacher who can be replaced by a machine deserves to be. Indeed, the computer will have considerably *less* effect on teachers than did the book, which destroyed the teacher's monopoly on knowledge, giving students the power, for the first time, to learn in private—and to learn as much as, or more than, their masters. The teaching technologies under development will change the teacher's role and function rather than diminish his importance.

Far from dehumanizing the learning process, in fact, computers and other electronic and mechanical aids are likely to *increase* the contact between students and teachers. By taking over much—perhaps most—of the rote and drill that now occupy teachers' time, the new technological devices will free teachers to do the kinds of things only human beings can do, playing the role of catalyst in group discussions and spending far more time working with students individually or in small groups. In short, the teacher will become a diagnostician, tutor, and Socratic leader rather than a drillmaster—the role he or she is usually forced to play today.

## The Decentralization of Knowledge

In the long run, moreover, the new information and teaching technologies will greatly accelerate the decentralization of knowledge and of education that began with the book. Because of television and the mass media, not to mention the incredible proliferation of education and training courses conducted by business firms and the armed forces, the schools are already beginning to lose their copyright on the word education. We are, as Cremin demonstrated in *The Genius of American Education,* returning to the classic Platonic and Jeffersonian concepts of education as a process carried on by the citizen's participation in the life of his community. At the very least, the schools will have to take account of the fact that students learn outside school as well as (and perhaps as much as) in school. Schools will, in consequence, have to start concentrating on the things they can teach best.

New pedagogies and new technologies will drastically alter the internal organization of the school as well as its relation to other educational institutions. Present methods of grouping a school population by grade and class, and present methods of organization within the individual classroom, are incompatible with any real emphasis on individual differences in learning. In the short run, this incompatibility may tend to defeat efforts to individualize instruction. But in the long run, the methods of school and classroom organization will have to accommodate themselves to what education will demand.

In the end, what education will demand will depend on what Americans, as a society, demand of it—which is to say, on the value we place on knowledge and its development. The potential seems clear enough. From the standpoint of what people are already capable of learning, we are all "culturally deprived"—and new knowledge about learning and new teaching technologies will expand our capacity to learn by several orders of magnitude. "Our chief want in life," Emerson wrote, "is someone who will make us do what we can."

# BIBLIOGRAPHY

An asterisk (*) preceding a reference indicates that the article or a part of it has been reprinted in this book.

## Books, Pamphlets, and Documents

Adler, Irving. What we want of our schools; plain talk on education, from theory to budgets. Day. New York. '57.

Alcorn, M. D. and others. Better teaching in secondary schools. rev. ed. Holt. New York. '64.

Ashton-Warner, Sylvia. Teacher. Simon and Schuster. New York. '63.

Baker, H. J. Introduction to exceptional children. 3d ed. Macmillan. New York. '59.

Beauchamp, G. A. Curriculum of the elementary school. Allyn. Boston. '64.

Bent, R. K. and Kronenberg, H. H. Principles of secondary education. 4th ed. McGraw-Hill. New York. '61.

Black, Hillel. They shall not pass. Morrow. New York. '63.

Brickman, W. W. and Lehrer, Stanley, eds. Automation, education, and human values. School and Society Books. New York. '66.

Brown, B. F. Nongraded high school. Prentice-Hall. Englewood Cliffs, N.J. '63.

Brubacher, J. S. History of the problems of education. McGraw-Hill. New York. '66.

Bruner, J. S. Process of education. Harvard University Press. Cambridge, Mass. '60.

Bruner, J. S. Toward a theory of instruction. Harvard University Press. Cambridge, Mass. '66.
    Excerpts: Commentary. 41:41-6. F. '66; Saturday Review. 49:70-2+. F. 19, '66.

Buckley, I. P. College begins at two. Whiteside. New York. '65.

Campbell, R. F. and others. Organization and control of American schools. Merrill. Columbus, Ohio. '65.

Conant, J. B. American high school today. McGraw-Hill. New York. '59.

Conant, J. B. Comprehensive high school: a second report to interested citizens. McGraw-Hill. New York. '67.

Conant, J. B. Education and liberty; the role of the schools in a modern democracy. Harvard University Press. Cambridge, Mass. '53.

Conant, J. B. Education of American teachers. McGraw-Hill. New York. '63.

Conant, J. B. Shaping educational policy. McGraw-Hill. New York. '64.

Conant, J. B. Slums and suburbs; a commentary on schools in metropolitan areas. McGraw-Hill. New York. '61.

Cook, L. A. and Cook, E. F. Sociological approach to education. McGraw-Hill. New York. '60.

Cremin, L. A. Genius of American education. Vintage. New York. '66.

Cremin, L. A. Transformation of the school. Vintage. New York. '64.

Davis, F. B. ed. Modern educational developments: another look. Educational Records Bureau. 21 Audubon Ave. New York 10032. '66.

Dewey, John. Democracy and education; an introduction to the philosophy of education. Macmillan. New York. '26.

Doman, G. J. How to teach your baby to read; the gentle revolution. Random House. New York. '64.

Ebel, R. L. Measuring educational achievement. Prentice-Hall. Englewood Cliffs, N.J. '65.

Eble, K. E. Perfect education. Macmillan. New York. '66.

Engelmann, Siegfried and Engelmann, Therese. Give your child a superior mind; a program for the preschool child. Simon and Schuster. New York. '66.

Fenton, Edwin. Teaching the new social studies in secondary schools: an inductive approach. Holt. New York. '66.

Fine, Benjamin. Your child and school. Macmillan. New York. '65.

Fletcher, C. S. ed. Education: the challenge ahead. Norton. New York. '62.

French, W. M. America's educational tradition; an interpretive history. Heath. Boston. '64.

Friedenberg, E. Z. Coming of age in America: growth and acquiescence. Random House. New York. '65.

Gardner, J. W. Excellence: can we be equal and excellent too? Harper. New York. '61.

Gerberich, J. R. and others. Measurement and evaluation in the modern school. McKay. New York. '62.

Goodlad, J. I. and Anderson, R. H. Nongraded elementary school. rev. ed. Harcourt. '63.

Goodlad, J. I. and others. Changing school curriculum. Fund for the Advancement of Education. 477 Madison Ave. New York 10022.

Goodman, Paul. Compulsory mis-education. Horizon Press. New York. '64.

Grambs, J. D. Schools, scholars, and society. Prentice-Hall. Englewood Cliffs, N.J. '65.

Greeley, A. M. and Rossi, P. H. Education of American Catholics. Aldine Publishing Company. Chicago. '66.

Greene, M. F. and Ryan, Oleta. The schoolchildren. Pantheon. New York. '66.

Gross, Ronald and Murphy, Judith, eds. Revolution in the schools. Harcourt. New York. '64.

Gwynn, J. M. Curriculum principles and social trends. 3d ed. Macmillan. New York. '60.

Hanna, L. A. and others. Unit teaching in the elementary school; social studies and related sciences. rev. ed. Holt. New York. '63.

Hanna, P. R. ed. Education: an instrument of national goals; papers presented at 1961 Cubberley Conference, School of Education, Stanford University. McGraw-Hill. New York. '62.

Hawes, G. R. Educational testing for the millions; what tests really mean for your child. McGraw-Hill. New York. '64.

Hechinger, F. M. ed. Pre-school education today; new approaches to teaching three- , four- , and five-year olds. Doubleday. Garden City, N.Y. '66.

Hentoff, Nat. Our children are dying. Viking Press. New York. '66.

Hildebrand, J. H. Is intelligence important? Macmillan. New York. '63.

Hoffmann, Banesh. Tyranny of testing. Crowell. New York. '62.

Holt, J. C. How children fail. Pitman. New York. '64.

Jameson, M. C. Helping your child succeed in elementary school. Putnam. New York. '62.

Kaufman, Bel. Up the down staircase. Prentice-Hall. Englewood Cliffs, N.J. '64.

Kemeny, J. G. Random essays on mathematics, education and computers. Prentice-Hall. Englewood Cliffs, N.J. '64.

Keppel, Francis. Necessary revolution in American education. Harper. New York. '66.

Kerber, August and Bommarito, Barbara, eds. Schools and the urban crisis; a book of readings. Holt. New York. '65.

Kneller, G. F. ed. Foundations of education. Wiley. New York. '63.

Krug, E. A. Shaping of the American high school. Harper. New York. '64.

Lamb, Pose. Student teaching process in elementary schools. Merrill. Columbus, Ohio. '65.

Landes, Ruth. Culture in American education: anthropological approaches to minority and dominant groups in the schools. Wiley. New York. '65.

Langdon, Grace and Stout, I. W. Teaching in the primary grades. Macmillan. New York. '64.

Leonard, E. M. and others. Foundations of learning in childhood education. Merrill. Columbus, Ohio. '63.

Loretan, J. O. and Umans, Shelley. Teaching the disadvantaged; new curriculum approaches. Teachers College Press. New York. '66.

McClellan, G. S. ed. America's educational needs. (Reference Shelf. v 30, no 5) Wilson. New York. '58.

Mayer, Martin. The schools. Harper. New York. '61.

Montessori, Maria. Dr. Montessori's own handbook. Bentley. Cambridge, Mass. '65.
  First published by Stokes in 1914.

*Morse, A. D. Schools of tomorrow—today! Doubleday. Garden City, N.Y. '60.

National Committee for Support of the Public Schools. Education and social change. The Committee. 1424 16th St. N.W. Washington, D.C. 20036. '66.

National School Public Relations Association. Shape of education for 1966-67, vol. 8; a handbook on current educational affairs. The Association. 1201 16th St. N.W. Washington, D.C. 20036. '66.

Neuwien, R. A. ed. Catholic schools in action. University of Notre Dame Press. South Bend, Ind. '66.

Otto, H. J. Elementary school organization and administration. 4th ed. Appleton. New York. '64.

Passow, A. H. ed. Education in depressed areas. Teachers College Press. New York. '63.

Petersen, D. G. and Hayden, V. D. Teaching and learning in the elementary school. Appleton. New York. '61.

Rafferty, M. L. Suffer, little children. Devin-Adair. New York. '62.

Rafferty, M. L. What they are doing to your children. New American Library. New York. '64.

Raywid, M. A. Ax-grinders: critics of our public schools. Macmillan. New York. '62.

Rickover, H. G. American education, a national failure; the problem of our schools and what we can learn from England. Dutton. New York. '63.

Rickover, H. G. Education and freedom. Dutton. New York. '59.

Ryan, P. J. Historical foundations of public education in America. Wm. C. Brown. Dubuque, Iowa. '65.

Sanford, Terry. But what about the people? Harper. New York. '66.

Sarratt, Reed. Ordeal of desegregation; the first decade. Harper. New York. '66.

Schaefer, R. J. School as a center of inquiry. Harper. New York. '67.

Schrag, Peter. Voices in the classroom. Beacon Press. Boston. '65.

Sexton, P. C. Education and income; inequities of opportunity in our public schools. Viking Press. New York. '61.

Smith, H. F. Secondary school teaching; modes for reflective thinking. Wm. C. Brown. Dubuque, Iowa. '64.

Stanford University. Institute for Communication Research. Educational television; the next ten years [a report and summary of major studies on the problems and potential of educational television, conducted under the auspices of the U.S. Office of Education]. The Institute. Stanford, Calif. '62.

Steel, Ronald, ed. Federal aid to education. (Reference Shelf. v 33, no 4) Wilson. New York. '61.

Tanner, Daniel. Schools for youth; change and challenge in secondary education. Macmillan. New York. '65.

Thayer, V. T. Formative ideas in American education. Dodd. New York. '65.
    *Excerpt:* School and Society. 93:183-96. Mr. 20, '65. Relation of the school to the social order.

Thomas, R. B. Search for a common learning: general education, 1800-1960. McGraw-Hill. New York. '62.

Todd, V. E. and Heffernan, Helen. Years before school; guiding preschool children. Macmillan. New York. '64.

United Nations Economic and Social Council. International Conference on public education, XXVIIIth session 1965. (Pub. no 282) UNESCO Publications Center. Dept. WS. 319 E. 34th St. New York 10016. '65.

United States. Congress. Joint Economic Committee. Automation and technology in education; a report of the Subcommittee on Economic Progress. 89th Congress, 2d session. Supt. of Docs. Washington, D.C. 20402. '66.

United States. Department of Health, Education, and Welfare. Education Office. Contemporary issues in American education; consultants' papers prepared for use at the White House Conference on Education, July 20-21, 1965. Supt. of Docs. Washington, D.C. 20402. '65.

United States. Department of Health, Education, and Welfare. Education Office. Equality of educational opportunity; by J. S. Coleman [and others]. Supt. of Docs. Washington, D.C. 20402. '66.

United States. Department of Health, Education, and Welfare. Education Office. General statement of policies under title VI of Civil Rights Act of 1964 respecting desegregation of elementary and secondary schools. The Office. Washington, D.C. 20202. Ap. '65.

United States. Department of Health, Education, and Welfare. Education Office. Revised statement of policies for school desegregation plans under title VI of the Civil rights act of 1964. The Office. Washington, D.C. 20202. Mr. '66.

United States. President's Science Advisory Committee. Innovation and experiment in education; a progress report of the Panel on Educational Research and Development. Supt. of Docs. Washington, D.C. 20402. '64.

Van Doren, Mark. Liberal education. Beacon Press. Boston. '59.

Venn, Grant. Man, education and work. American Council on Education. 1785 Massachusetts Ave. N.W. Washington, D.C. 20036. '64.

### PERIODICALS

America. 112:512. Ap. 17, '65. New York textbook bill.

America. 112:553. Ap. 17, '65. Case for a narrow education. R. L. Dean.

America. 112:796. My. 29, '65. Aid for all; state to pay the full cost of textbooks in public schools.

*American Education. 1:13-20. Ap. '65. ". . . The first work of these times . . ."; a description and analysis of the Elementary and Secondary Education Act of 1965.

American Education. 1:1-3. Jl. '65. Big ideas for small schools. D. F. Parody.

American Education. 1:27. S. '65. Message from the President to all who work with youth. L. B. Johnson.

*American Education. 2:9-13. Je. '66. Lively third R. K. E. Brown and others.

*American Education. 2:inside front cover. S. '66. View from afar. Harold Howe II.

*American Education. 2:20-2. S. '66. Head Start or false start? C. S. Carleton.

American Education. 2:23. S. '66. Back-to-school statistics.

*American Education. 2:1-7. O. '66. How good are our schools? Richard de Neufville and Caryl Conner.

*American Education. 2:10-12. O. '66. From Maine to California: revolution in summer schools. B. H. Pearse.

Business Week. p 110-12. Ap. 10, '65. Spreading the word on the new math: use of telephone lines and the Electrowriter.

*Carnegie Quarterly. 14:1-3. Fall '66. Rich get richer & the poor get poorer . . . schools.

Changing Times. 19:32-4. Ag. '65. Teaching kids before they start school.

Changing Times. 20:24-9. Ja. '66. Doctor James B. Conant answers questions you ask about schools. J. B. Conant.

Changing Times. 20:6-10. S. '66. Are schools changing too much too fast?

Christian Century. 83:186-8. F. 9, '66. Searchlight on high schools in the South. W. W. Geier.

Christian Century. 83:234-5. F. 23, '66. State of Iowa vs. the Amish; school dispute. F. H. Littell.

Christian Century. 83:245-7. F. 23, '66. That Amish thing; education dispute in Iowa. P. B. Mather.

Christian Century. 83:474-6. Ap. 13, '66. Amish controversy; temporarily settled: Gov. Hughes acts. P. B. Mather.

Christian Century. 83:862-4. Jl. 6, '66. Art, technology and education; excerpt from address, February 1966. A. I. Cox, Jr.

Clearing House. 40:532-7. My. '66. Rise and fall of the core curriculum. Harvey Overton.
> *Same condensed:* Education Digest. 32:45-8. O. '66.

Commonweal. 81:595-6. F. 5, '65. Money from heaven? question of spending so much for science.

Commonweal. 81:638-40. F. 12, '65. Johnson education bill. W. B. Ball.

Education. 86:221-5. D. '65. New programs race. C. O. Olson, Jr.

Education. 87:37-41. S. '66. Teaching reading to young children. Dolores Durkin.

Education Digest. 30:22-4. My. '65. Team teaching in the high school. C. H. Peterson.

Education Digest. 31:8-11. Ja. '66. Principles of school desegregation. H. O. Hall and D. L. Leonard.

Education Digest. 32:22-5. S. '66. Secondary education tomorrow. J. L. Trump.

Elementary School Journal. 65:300-5. Mr. '65. Are kindergartens obsolete? Bernard Spodek and H. F. Robison.
> *Same condensed:* Education Digest. 31:19-21. S. '65.

*Fortune. 74:120-5+. Ag. '66. Technology is knocking at the schoolhouse door. C. E. Silberman.

Good Housekeeping. 160:132-3. Ja. '65. New math your children may be learning.

Good Housekeeping. 162:138. Ja. '66. School enrichment; what it is and is not.

*Harper's Magazine. 226:33-40. Ap. '63. Learning to be unemployable. E. T. Chase.

*Harper's Magazine. 229:82-4+. O. '64. Coming revolution in teaching English. Andrew Schiller.

Harper's Magazine. 231:134-7. S. '65. Understanding the new math? Darrell Huff.

Harper's Magazine. 232:102-3. My. '66. On schools: are the children in the running? John Holt.

Harvard Education Review. 36:284-94. Summer '66. Effect of segregation on the aspirations of Negro youth. N. H. St. John.

High School Journal. 49:1-5. O. '65. Chaos in the social studies. D. W. Robinson.

Illinois Education. 54:62-7. O. '65. Giving them a head start. Francine Richard.
    *Same condensed:* Education Digest. 31:21-4. Ja. '66.

Instructor. 75:24+. Ja. '66. Inquiry in the curriculum. J. R. Suchman.

Instructor. 76:146. N. '66. Individualizing the primary program. Lena Maxwell.

Intercom. 8:18-23. N.-D. '66. Memo to teachers; technology and teaching: the new partnership.

Journal of Negro Education. 34:232-3. Summer '65. Legislation and its implementation; the South. J. A. Morsell.

Journal of Negro Education. 34:258-67. Summer '65. Community behavior and northern school desegregation. R. A. Dentler.

Journal of Negro Education. 34:310-18. Summer '65. Programs in the South. E. H. West and W. G. Daniel.

Journal of Negro Education. 35:55-61. Winter '66. Comparative study of selected perceptions and feelings of Negro adolescents with and without white friends in integrated urban high schools. S. W. Webster and M. N. Kroger.

Library Journal. 90:1999-2000. Ap. 15, '65. Humanities in the ninth grade introduced in project Cue.

Look. 30:100+. My. 17, '66. What better schools will cost [interviews ed. by S. Wren]. J. W. Gardner.

McCall's. 92:94. F. '65. How much have our schools improved since sputnik? questions and answers. Grace Hechinger and F. M. Hechinger.

Michigan Education Journal. 43:18-19. Mr. '66. Many things are right with U.S. public schools. Ute Auld.

Monthly Labor Review. 88:625-8. Je. '65. Rising levels of education among young workers. J. D. Cowhig and C. L. Beale.

NEA Journal. 54:28-30+. F. '65. Mathematics for the low achiever. Irving Adler.

NEA Journal. 54:46-7. N. '65. Breakthrough for professional autonomy; status of teaching profession in Oregon. E. S. Crowley.

NEA Journal. 54:30-2. D. '65. Sharing good teaching practices. R. O. Lippitt and M. P. Flanders.

NEA Journal. 55:33-7. F. '66. Educational opportunity around the world.

NEA Journal. 55:30-2. Mr. '66. What educational plan for the in-between-ager? the six-three-three plan and others. W. M. Alexander.

NEA Journal. 55:27-8+. Ap. '66. Regional approaches to educational problems. P. F. Johnston.

NEA Journal. 55:33-5. Ap. '66. Roots of failure. K. C. Cotter.
    *Discussion:* Elementary school comment. p 35-6. M. W. Hass; Secondary school comment. p 36. J. E. Mizer.

NEA Journal. 55:13-14. S. '66. Culturally disadvantaged children can be helped. Lessie Carlton and R. H. Moore.

Nation's Business. 53:27-8. F. '65. Education's faceless factories short-change our students. Felix Morley.

Nation's Schools. 77:71+. F. '66. Courts rule both ways on *de facto* segregation L. O. Garber.

Nation's Schools. 77:32. Mr. '66. Help us over the desegregation hump. D. S. Seeley.

Nation's Schools. 77:70-3. Ap. '66. What's happening in curriculum development. J. I. Goodlad and M. F. Klein.

Nation's Schools. 77:48-9+. Je. '66. Preprimary programs; will public schools control Head Start? Erwin Knoll.

Nation's Schools. 78:48. Ag. '66. Are you sure pupils are better off at school? how to help hard-core delinquents. Arthur Pearl.

Nation's Schools. 78:10+. S. '66. Let's not force preschool programs on everybody. A. H. Rice.

*New Republic. 152:17-20. F. 6, '65. LBJ's school program: a revolution in American education? Christopher Jencks.

New Republic. 153:5-6. O. 9, '65. Black and white schools; separate and unequal schools in the South.

New Republic. 154:8-9. Ap. 9, '66. Forcing desegregation through Title VI; new guidelines. A. M. Bickel.
    *Reply:* 154:29-30. Ap. 23, '66. C. White.

New Republic. 155:21-6. O. 1, '66. Education: the racial gap; findings of James Coleman's study. Christopher Jencks.

New York Times. p 53. F. 5, '67. Sweeping changes in Catholic schools urged by educator at Notre Dame. Gene Currivan.

New York Times. p E7. Mr. 5, '67. Conant: a new report by the schools' Mr. Fixit. F. M. Hechinger.

New York Times. p 1+. Mr. 7, '67. U.S. ranked low in math teaching. F. M. Hechinger.

New York Times Magazine. p 46-7+. My. 1, '66. Fourth R, the rat race; schools as high-pressure learning factories. John Holt.

Newsweek. 65:112+. My. 10, '65. New math: does it really add up?

Newsweek. 65:64. My. 24, '65. Subminimal Oklahoma; NEA imposes sanctions because of bad academic conditions.

Newsweek. 66:19-20. S. 6, '65. Year of compliance.

Newsweek. 66:65. D. 13, '65. Toward the new South; Southern region conference.

PTA Magazine. 60:8-10, 36. O. '65. Adding up the new math; with study-discussion program by Elizabeth Harris and Dale Harris. Patrick Suppes.

PTA Magazine. 60:2-3. N. '65. Capital gains. Jennelle Moorhead.

PTA Magazine. 60:4-7, 34-5. N. '65. Education: what kind, for whom, how much? with study-discussion program by Carol Smallenburg and Harry Smallenburg. G. L. Mangum.

PTA Magazine. 60:14. D. '65. What's happening in education? Middle schools. W. D. Boutwell.

PTA Magazine. 60:13-14. F. '66. What's happening in education? Interstate program for cooperation on educational problems. W. D. Boutwell.

PTA Magazine. 60:2-3. Mr. '66. Who's blocking educational change? excerpts from address. Jennelle Moorhead.

*PTA Magazine. 60:18-21. Ap. '66. Coming revolution against boredom in the classroom. J. N. Miller.
    Same condensed with title: New cure for boredom in the classroom. Reader's Digest. 88:171-2+. My. '66.

Parents' Magazine. 41:26, 52-3+. Mr. '66. School system that failed; with discussion group program, by M. S. Smart. William Hartley and Ellen Hartley.

Parents' Magazine. 41:30. Ap. '66. Challenge to our schools. J. H. Fischer.

Parents' Magazine. 41:52. S. '66. Meeting our educational needs. J. H. Fischer.

Phi Delta Kappan. 46:481. Je. '65. Are national achievement testing and a national curriculum coming?

Phi Delta Kappan. 47:254-7. Ja. '66. Federal courts and racial imbalance in public schools. S. F. Roach.

Phi Delta Kappan. 47:258-62. Ja. '66. Can team teaching save the core curriculum? G. F. Vars.

Phi Delta Kappan. 47:301-4. F. '66. Modern functional adaptations to the abler student. H. R. Douglass.

*Phi Delta Kappan. 47:482-6. My. '66. Civil rights fiasco in public education. Myron Lieberman.
    *Same:* Teachers College Record. 68:120-6. N. '66.

Phi Delta Kappan. 47:515-17. My. '66. Redefining of rights. S. S. Shermis.

Phi Delta Kappan. 48:62-4. O. '66. Whatever happened to the ideal of the comprehensive school? D. U. Levine.

*Public Interest. p 59-69. Summer '66. Search for "brainpower." G. C. Keller.

*Public Interest. p 70-5. Summer '66. Equal schools or equal students? J. S. Coleman.

Publishers' Weekly. 188:13-27, 40. N. 1, '65. Role of paperback books in education examined in depth; summary of conference at Teachers College, Columbia University; with editorial comment.

Reader's Digest. 86:78-82. F. '65. New careers in America's classrooms. Lester Velie.

Redbook. 125:58-9+. My. '65. Best weapon in the fight for better education; question of school boards and quality of schools. Bernard Asbell.

Redbook. 125:26+. O. '65. Why I don't believe in speeding up primary education. Benjamin Spock.

Redbook. 126:8+. Mr. '66. Segregation fence: a young mother gets involved. Mary Jaynes.

Reporter. 33:31-3. Ag. 12, '65. Integrating the Negro teacher out of a job; dilemma in Munday. Barbara Carter.
    *Discussion:* 33:10+. S. 23, '65.

Reporter. 33:34-7. S. 9, '65. Teachers give Oklahoma a lesson; NEA sanctions against state. Barbara Carter.

Reporter. 34:34. Ja. 13, '66. Will evolution come to Arkansas? Tom Dearmore.

Saturday Review. 48:56-7+. Ja. 16, '65. How sinister is the education establishment? D. W. Robinson.
    *Reply:* 48:96. F. 20, '65. M. E. Doyle.

Saturday Review. 48:84-5. F. 20, '65. Full educational opportunity; key points of President's message. L. B. Johnson.

Saturday Review. 48:60-1+. Mr. 20, '65. Title VI: southern education faces the facts; guidelines to school authorities. G. W. Foster, Jr.

Saturday Review. 48:62-3+. Mr. 20, '65. Progress report on the mathematics revolution. Evelyn Sharp.

Saturday Review. 48:66-7. Mr. 20, '65. Transatlantic view of American education. Monroe Whitney.

Saturday Review. 48:55-6+. Je. 19, '65. Organizing for continuing change. F. A. Ianni and B. D. McNeill.

Saturday Review. 48:62-3. Jl. 17, '65. Do-it-yourself in Granby; experiment to improve educational opportunities. E. D. Stevens.

Saturday Review. 48:53. Ag. 21, '65. Faddishness in education. Mortimer Smith.

Saturday Review. 48:66-7+. S. 11, '65. Are we educating our children for the wrong future? R. M. Hutchins.

Saturday Review. 48:80-1+. O. 16, '65. Why teachers fail; address. B. F. Skinner.

Saturday Review. 48:88. O. 16, '65. What's bugging teachers. A. M. West.

Saturday Review. 48:89-90+. O. 16, '65. Do school boards take education seriously? John Wallace and Phillip Schneider.

Saturday Review. 48:62+. D. 18, '65. Head Start in suburbia; Yorktown, Westchester County. Jill Nagy.

Saturday Review. 49:88. Ap. 16, '66. Who pulled the teeth from Title VI? G. W. Foster, Jr.

Saturday Review. 49:89. Ap. 16, '66. We thought they meant it; actions against Negroes enrolling their children in previously all-white schools.

Saturday Review. 49:71-2. S. 17, '66. National assessment; Exploratory committee on assessing the progress of education. Paul Woodring.

*Saturday Review. 49:72-4+. O. 15, '66. Catholics and their schools. John Cogley.

Saturday Review. 49:75. O. 15, '66. Magnitude of the American educational establishment (1966-1967).

Saturday Review. 49:80-1+. O. 15, '66. History and the new social studies. R. H. Brown.

Saturday Review. 49:87. O. 15, '66. Is there a new establishment? Peter Schrag.

School and Society. 93:147-50. Mr. 6, '65. Educational values in disorder. Joseph Justman.

School and Society. 93:175-7. Mr. 20, '65. Excellence in education: foundation of the Great Society; excerpt from address, November 24, 1964. H. H. Humphrey.

School and Society. 93:252-4. Ap. 17, '65. Recent developments in mathematics education. H. E. Bowie.

School and Society. 93:388. O. 30, '65. Educating Spanish-speaking children.

School and Society. 93:429-30. N. 13, '65. Education is for thinking. R. D. Patton.

School and Society. 93:474-5. D. 11, '65. Dichotomies in American education. J. J. Van Patten.

School and Society. 93:491-2. D. 25, '65. Education in 1965; major educational events. W. W. Brickman.

School and Society. 94:67. F. 5, '66. 1966 as a centennial year in the history of education. Franklin Parker.

School and Society. 94:171-2. Ap. 2, '66. Faults and hopeful signs in education.

School and Society. 94:183-4. Ap. 2, '66. High school in the South.

Science. 153:1197. S. 9, '66. Preschool education. L. N. Morrisett.

Science. 153:1624-6. S. 30, '66. Technology in the schools; educators are uneasy. L. J. Carter.

Science News Letter. 87:70. Ja. 30, '65. More education needed.

Senior Scholastic. 86:14T. F. 4; sup 3. My. 20; 87:sup 3. O. 14, '65. Washington report. John Lloyd.

Senior Scholastic. 86:sup 10-11. Mr. 25, '65. New era in Michigan education. L. M. Bartlett.

Senior Scholastic. 87:sup 16-17. O. 14, '65. Innovations in foreign language instruction. T. T. Ladu.

Senior Scholastic. 87:sup 21-2. O. 28, '65. Paperbacks on the march; concerning paperbound books in New Jersey public schools. Max Bogart.

Senior Scholastic. 87:sup 22-3. O. 28, '65. Profile of a high school; New Jersey paperback study.

Senior Scholastic. 87:sup 2. Ja. 7, '66. Compact plan moves toward ratification: nationwide policy for education.

Senior Scholastic. 88:sup 7. F. 4; sup 8. F. 11, '66. Washington report; concerning the report, Local school expenditures: 1970 projections.

Senior Scholastic. 89:sup 13. O. 7, '66. Education and the new technology; symposium.

Teachers College Record. 67:18-25. O. '65. Balance in high school education. H. J. Klausmeier.

Teachers College Record. 68:61-4. O. '66. Risks of initiative. M. Greene.

Time. 85:49-50. Mr. 19, '65. Catching failures in time; costly public boarding school in Winston-Salem for underachievers.

Time. 85:58+. Je. 18, '65. Segregation by integration; problem of Negro teachers.

Time. 86:56. Ag. 27, '65. Another first for Massachusetts; ban de facto school segregation.

Time. 87:51. Je. 3, '66. How parents feel; survey of attitudes toward schools, made for the Charles F. Kettering foundation.

Time. 88:39. Jl. 1, '66. School for four-year-olds?

Time. 88:44-5. Ag. 12, '66. Teaching baby to read.

Time. 88:100. O. 21, '66. Shadow schools; academic undergrounds.

U.S. News & World Report. 58:54. My. 3, '65. Shared time in action, case history; Cheboygan, Mich.

U.S. News & World Report. 58:16. My. 24, '65. Behind a controversy over pay for teachers.

*U.S. News & World Report. 58:53-6. Je. 14, '65. One campus for all schools—is this your city's solution?

U.S. News & World Report. 59:6. S. 6, '65. In school this autumn: more than a fourth of U.S. population.

U.S. News & World Report. 59:40. S 13, '65. Integration takes hold in southern schools.

U.S. News & World Report. 59:44-7. S. 27, '65. Big-city schools in trouble? resegregation in North.

*U.S. News & World Report. 60:52-4+. F. 21, '66. Forgotten youth in today's America.

*U.S. News & World Report. 61:49-50. S. 5, '66. Is Federal aid helping to end neighborhood schools?

Vital Speeches of the Day. 31:307-10. Mr. 1, '65. Metropolitan education; address, January 27, 1965. R. M. Besse.

Vital Speeches of the Day. 32:275-8. F. 15, '66. Education without magic; address, November 19, 1965. J. M. Moudy.

Wilson Library Bulletin. 39:860-6. Je. '65. South: educational resources; address, April 1965. Reed Sarratt.